Medical Axioms: 1st Edition

Up to about October 2014 or so
Updated with corrections 2/15/2018

Mark B. Reid, MD
Internal Medicine Hospitalist
Denver, Colorado

On Twitter @medicalaxioms
Email: medicalaxioms@gmail.com

Acknowledgments

I'd like to thank my Special Lady Friend Kate for her support and guidance through the last three years of this project. I am by nature full of good ideas and more prone to start projects than to finish them. She has supplied the necessary focus and support to allow me to do something I've never actually done before—finish a project. Her calm good judgment and level-headed support has made this whole thing possible. At the same time, she always makes everything sporty and fun, reminds me to go outside and play, enjoys a good fit of brainstorming and daydreaming, and is pretty to look at. Thank you, Kate!

As any of you who follow me on Twitter @medicalaxioms know, these aphorisms are hardly generated in a vacuum. There is a constant interplay between me and all the people nice enough to read my free flow sometimes stream-of-consciousness banter. I generate a heap of chaff in the process of trying to get a bag of grain and the readers help me with the sorting, correct my tone, point me in new directions and all kinds of good stuff. In the Second Edition, I hope to include more of your edits and aphorisms, attributed.

About this Book: Disclaimer

I never wrote a book before and I couldn't find anyone to publish this one so I did it myself. That being said, I don't know anything about book-making. The book may have problems. There may be typos and the format might be off, especially if you are reading the first edition. You might not like some words and some aphorisms may irk you. Apologies beforehand. If you really want to be helpful, feel free to suggest edits to me by email at medicalaxioms@gmail.com. If you find two identical aphorisms, feel free to identify them by number and text and send your discovery to me. I'd really appreciate it and it would make the next edition better.

In my own life, I have found it very liberating to move away from criticism and toward *offering suggestions for improvement.* I do this in my home life and in the hospital and I find it is often appreciated as I am taking on some of the work to make the thing better, myself.

About the Author

I am not a real author or anything. In fact, throughout my life I have had problems with reading and writing. So in medical school I had to squash complicated concepts into short sentences and write things repeatedly to learn them. This has generally been a liability but a tolerable necessity as a slow learner. Until the social media came along. Twitter's original 140 character limit was a perfect match for the length of writing I could read or produce. A fortunate coincidence that has resulted in this book!

I was born in Cincinnati Ohio the youngest of 4 kids. My parents were a physicist turned industrial manager and a genius geologist turned housewife. They supplied a lot of good books about science for me specifically a series of Time Life picture books and let me build a chemistry lab in the furnace room, experiment with fire and electricity, and generally enjoyed my eccentricities.

After a brief period of delinquency in 8th grade, I attended St. Xavier High School and credit the Jesuits with fixing about ½ of what was wrong with me. I still abide by their motto "Men for others." I got into Williams College as a legacy and proceeded to row on the crew team, build a bicycle team, and generally not deliver at the level of my academic potential. There was no better place on earth to do that than with a bunch of smart overachievers in Williamstown, MA.

Upon graduation, I lived on a guy's couch in Washington, DC, became a bicycle messenger then ambulance driver then rat murderer in a lab at GW then an eyeball dissector and HPLC operator at the NEI at the NIH. Case Western Reserve University was the only medical school that would have me and they formed the fundamentals of my approach to teaching medicine that I present to you here.

I did my internship and residency in Internal Medicine with Bob Schrier, MD at the University of Colorado in Denver. This was an amazing program—huge and diverse with a University Hospital, VA, county and 2 private hospitals. I learned so much I had to study very little for boards. I answered every question by recalling a case I had seen. I had a wonderful diversity of clinical educators and borrowed many tricks and styles from them. Then I was a chief resident and went into private practice for a few years until Rick K. Albert, MD invited me back to join a newly formed hospitalist group at Denver Health Medical Center where I have remained since.

I have two talented and fascinating genius daughters, a whip-smart Lady Friend with two brilliant daughters of her own, a top-notch cattle dog and a committee of dedicated friends who keep me out of trouble, usually.

—Mark

Table of Contents:

Foreword

After following Mark on social media for many years, I was delighted to learn he was planning to publish a compendium of his many remarkable tweets. I have known Mark for over twenty years and watched him grow from a rookie house officer to an attending physician and now to a master clinician. Above all, he is a kind, gifted physician with the ability to see the best in people, learn from others even under the most difficult situations and deliver kindness and humor when many of us would have complained and whined. The collection of tweets in this volume is really the best of Mark Reid. He is witty, concise yet thoughtful, kind, humorous. The brief tweets he labels as Medical Axioms are wise and inspirational. Read when you need a pick me up or just when you need to be assured that you are headed in the right direction in your own world.

Stu Linas, MD
Professor, Medicine-Renal Med Diseases/Hypertension
Chief of Nephrology, Department of Medicine
University of Colorado Hospital
Denver Health Medical Center

Note from the Author

In writing these aphorisms since 2010, I discovered the inherent value in this system of capturing truth. No aphorism is true all the time in any circumstances. Good ones are often or usually true and easy to remember. Then their few exceptions can also be committed to memory. *There is no more efficient way to capture human wisdom than to learn a rule and its exceptions.*

The aphorisms contained in this book are not universally true. Every one of them has exceptions. As you read, these will come to mind. As a critical thinker, you will say "Not always!" and "I know an exception!" This is understood and expected. That dialogue between us is essential. This project has always been interactive. If you have a correction or note an error, please email me directly at medicalaxioms@gmail.com or tweet your improvement to my words on Twitter @medicalaxioms. I by no means have access to truth. I only seek truth. You, too, are a truth seeker and I welcome your progress towards and understanding of the patient, the disease, and the healer and their interactions together.

In the end my message is simple and highly repetitive:

- Remember why you first signed up to be a medical person in the first place
- Remember your patient is sick and scared and you are here to help
- Keep learning. Keep teaching.
- Above all, inspire!

Teaching someone something is like driving a nail into a board. *Repetition is the foundation of learning.*

You'd think it would go without saying that the words in this book are not medical advice. But let me be very direct: These axioms are not medical advice. The practice of medicine requires an agreement between physician and patient to enter into a relationship that implies duty and trust between them. I don't have that relationship with readers of this book. Neither can medical judgment be kept in the confines of a book jacket. The practice of medicine requires book learning, closely-supervised training during the residency, ongoing professional study to keep up with changes in the literature, and the experience of practice—successes and failures that modify the way a physician treats the next patient they see. Some of these aphorisms conflict with one another and others are frankly contradictory. So is the practice of medicine. The treatment that can save one patient may kill another. A book that would allow the lay reader to know the difference would be a hundred feet thick and would need to be updated hourly.

Lastly, I hope this book inspires you as I have been inspired by other writers (see the final chapter of this book). If you feel inspired, tweet @medicalaxioms on Twitter and I will see it or if you prefer email me at medicalaxioms@gmail.com. I hope future editions of this book will contain attributed quotes from readers like you!

Mark B. Reid, MD
Internal Medicine Hospitalist
Denver, Colorado
On Twitter @medicalaxioms
medicalaxioms@gmail.com

General Principles

1. No rule is true in every case. Learning a rule and its exceptions offers the most efficient means of mastering the complexity of medicine.

2. When in doubt, save the life and apologize for saving the life afterwards.

3. The sickest patients do not get to pick their doctor. It is your responsibility to be competent.

4. Don't believe what you hear. Believe what you read. Medicine is full of hearsay, legend, and rumor. [This book is no different]

5. Medicine is a description of nature. Not a script for nature.

6. The next case might not look like the last one. Diseases present as differently as caterpillars and butterflies.

7.   When given a choice between knowing and not knowing, choose knowing.

8.   You are more likely to do wise things if you can say wise things.

9.   Your chance of making a good decision is improved if you can explain to someone how you made it.

10. Walking into a patient's room without at least glancing at the chart beforehand is like petting a dog you don't know.

11. Easy cases are easy. Use them to prepare for the hard cases.

12. More patients want their doctors to be gods than doctors think they are.

13. Recipe for Success: Stop doing the 95% of things that are never going to work. Put that effort toward the 5% that have a chance.

14. A complication in a live guy is better than no complication in a dead guy.

15. Over-prepare for complications that never occur.

16. You can't listen while talking.

17. Know your Three Primary Duties to your Patients:
    1) Diagnose and treat
    2) Reduce suffering
    3) Prevent disease

18. There are no rules in Medicine. Without rules, Medicine would be unteachable and unlearnable.

19. If you walk in the room and find the patient cold, hungry, or in pain, fix it immediately. They'll forever associate your face with the relief of suffering.

20. The most expensive test in the hospital is another hospital day. Except an exploratory laparotomy.

21. The number one cause of weight loss is "there is no weight loss." Figure out if the patient has truly lost weight before you go working it up!

22. The fish swims through water with the head in front and body following behind. Humans recover from illness the same.

23. God works in mysterious ways. Other times you will have to consult your doctor.

24. Insecurity is the foundation of ego. Humility is the foundation of confidence.

25. Life is short. Try not to make it any shorter than it was meant to be.

26. No diagnosis is wrong until it is replaced by a better one.

27. Like your dumb old parents, dumb old doctors get smarter as you get older.

28. Hard work on this side of the grave can save a life. On the other side, hard work results in a pretty flower arrangement at the funeral parlor.

29. Intravenous Catheter (n.): An invitation to Staph aureus to come vacation in your patient's normally sterile innards.

30. In order to return a sick patient to health, the physician must be able to envision the patient well again.

31. If you don't bring your humanity with you to work, you might have trouble finding it on your way home.

32. Wisdom is the offspring of Error and Humility.

33. With sufficient lack of preparation, even the easiest plans can go badly.

34. Good bedside manners are essential but the greatest kindness you can show your patient is competence.

35. Tolerance of mediocrity will get you more mediocrity.

36. I question the good sense of anyone who never ignores their doctor.

37. If all your patients hate you, they are probably right. If none of your patients hate you, you are probably doing something wrong.

38. There is no medicine that can replace the many benefits of having the obligations and responsibilities of a job.

39. Every patient with hemophilia and every IV drug addict knows the location of their last accessible vein. They just don't want to tell you.

40. I'm always surprised by the woman who is surprised by her newly discovered pregnancy.

41. Greatness is better achieved by the continuous application of gentle pressure than by any use of heroic effort.

42. As you gain knowledge and ex.
    become rare. Rarer.

43. You must monitor yourself closely at the e
    day, end of shift, end of week, end of rotatio.
    end of residency. Those are the times you'll
    make the most mistakes.

44. Complications sleep by day and prey at night.

45. Your patient is not your enemy.

46. There is no five-second rule in the hospital.

47. People revered doctors more when we had less
    to offer. We had to make up with compassion
    what we couldn't offer in treatment.

48. Nothing in medicine is always or never. Instead
    say these words: Usually, sometimes, often,
    rarely, and it depends.

.   When possible, make important decisions in the light of day. Plan for things that may go wrong in the dark of night.

50.   The human GI tract is like an old PC. If it's not working, turn it off, wait awhile, and turn it back on.

51.   Good medicine is good acting.

52.   Even when you feel certain you can outrun him, never give Death a head start.

53.   Frustrate Death with your:
      • Attention to changes
      • Systematic discipline
      • Calm

54.   The patient who needs your help the most can't ask for help.

55.   The second worst thing is knowing your patient has a terrible illness and is going to die. The worst thing is not knowing.

56. All gradually progressive illnesses are noticed suddenly.

57. Everybody lies to cops. The less you act like a cop, the less you will get lied to.

58. Never be a VIP. They get "special care" that deviates from standard care. All deviations from standard care are sub-standard.

59. Heroism is necessitated by poor planning.

60. Don't take advice about surviving at sea from someone who has never fallen off a boat.

61. Like toothpaste, blood is hard to get back in once it is out.

62. If you can't say it, you can't do it. You'll learn to say it by teaching it. Then you can do it!

63. There is no health in the body while there are bad teeth in the mouth.

64. The fewer the words, the greater the truth.

65. When you don't know something, look it up. It's a habit you'll use less and less.

66. Don't trust everything you hear from another doctor. Also, don't ignore anything you hear from another doctor.

67. Every day a patient spends in the hospital bed takes a week to recover.

68. All patients who take their medicines exactly as prescribed are liars.

69. A mediocre doctor standing in front of you is better than a great one asleep in her bed.

70. Even the best doctors make mistakes. Only the best doctors want to hear about them

71. Ninety percent of good medicine is good habits. Two percent is extremely challenging, creative problem solving. The rest is dumb luck.

72. The first hospital day is the riskiest. Over subsequent days, wrong hypotheses are destroyed by facts and time.

73. On success and failure:
    - Celebrate your successes—small compensation for your hard work.
    - Cherish your mistakes. They can make you great.

74. If you want medical people to be good, treat them with respect. If you want them to be great, feed them donuts.

75. Patients complain most about doctors who don't listen. Then doctors that don't talk.

76. You know who comes in your house and never takes a seat? The police. Don't stand around like a bunch of cops in the patient's room.

77. The further into the future we ask medicine to predict, the less accurate and more expensive it becomes.

78. Untreated hypertension leads to heart attacks and strokes. Likewise, untreated depression leads to suicides.

79. How come some doctors have such wonderful and appreciative patients? They make them.

80. If the next upward titration of any therapy should be done in the ICU then the patient should already be there.

81. Spend one minute making your plan and one more figuring out what to do if it doesn't work.

82. The best recipe to help yourself: Help patients and their families. Then colleagues, students, and nurses. Help your own family and friends. Help a complete stranger. Now you're helped.

83. Patients on heparin have DVTs; beta blockers MI; pneumonia vaccine get pneumonia. Prophylaxis, secondary prevention and vaccination improve the odds and sometimes lessen the severity. They don't always prevent the event.

84. If you go back to see a patient after you have gone off service, it is called a social call. Don't read the chart or look at the monitor. You aren't a doctor to a patient. You're a friend calling on a sick person.

85. A good doctor is at least as good as a good waiter—good natured, well-mannered, and efficient. Without being pushy.

86. Many patients feel better a day or two after they stop all their medicines.

87. A healthy person put in a hospital bed for a week will get sick with something.

88. In medicine it takes about as long to get well as it took to get sick. Not true in trauma surgery or OB.

89. Many mistakes in medicine can be remedied after they are identified. A poor first impression is not one of them.

90. Good patients are made, not found.

91. Much medical wisdom is neither evidence-based nor testable but it still works. When evidence proves a wives' tale wrong, abandon it remorseless.

92. They don't pay doctors enough to worry about their patients at home. Make decisions that you can leave in the hospital and clinic.

93. Never make decisions until necessary. Once committed, watch for signs of error. Abandon bad decisions in face of new evidence. — @cwrightmd

94. Two rules for any emergency:
    1. Don't lose your head.
    2. Don't die.

95. The key to getting people to help you is to be as helpful as possible.

96. Two patients died who changed my practice forever: My mom and dad. Neither was my patient.

97. Most doctors have a pretty good sense of how much various injuries and ailments hurt which is totally wrong.

98. Most doctors have a pretty good sense of how long it takes to get better from common surgeries and illnesses, which is totally wrong.

99. Sometimes when the old lady stops eating she's going to die soon and there is nothing you can do about it.

100. Put small effort into easy things. Save big efforts for big things.

101. Although you look better when you make a mistake by ignoring your gut and following the wrong advice of a subspecialist, you won't feel better.

102. The patient in front of you does not have "a 90% mortality." Their mortality is either 100% or 0%. Do your best and leave room for a miracle.

103. To navigate the patient's course in the hospital, keep 3 stars in view:
    1. Diagnosis + treatment
    2. Feelings of patient + family
    3. Alleviation of suffering.

104. No patient wants a hurried doctor—speed up between patients and slow down with them.

105. Try repeating this mantra with patients and staff: "Why are we here? To save some lives!" Or do what I do and repeat it to yourself as you walk into work every morning.

106. Relax your judgmental mind that knows who will die and when. Leave room for a miracle.

107. Anemia is usually missing blood. Don't stop until you find the blood.

108. If water is going in the vein and not coming out in the urine, find the water.

109. The practice of medicine—when done to excess and to the exclusion of other things—can lose its blessing and become a curse.

110. If you want things to go your way, bring pie.

111. A surprise anticipated is unsurprising.

112. Mediocre decisions made early outperform perfect decisions, late.

113. You know that feeling when something goes horribly wrong and you feel like you've been dunked in ice water and tossed onto an arctic glacier when you realize your mistake? We all know that feeling.

114. When a patient is repeatedly admitted to hospital and found to have "nothing wrong with them," ask them, "What are you looking for here?"

115. Fifty percent of your success comes from the last 10% of your effort. 10% from the last 1%.

116. The Three A's of Medicine, in order of perceived importance: "Affability, Availability, and Ability."
—Alex Bibbey, MD

117. The problem is not that doctors think they are gods. The problem is that some patients expect us to be.

118. All difficult medical decisions should be converted into multiple choice questions.

119. You spend the first ten years in medical practice mastering your rightness. The rest of your career is spent overcoming your wrongness.

120. One of the mysteries of modern medicine is how badly some people want to be doctors and how badly some doctors wish they were something else.

121. Close the door to the patient's room and leave the insurance companies and bureaucrats outside. Enjoy the quiet of a sick person in need of help and you able to deliver it.

122. The most beautiful medicine is seen by only two people.

123. Know your Achilles heel. Mine is sputum.

124. In the end, god leads all his little sheep back to the green meadow. Sometimes we hold tight to the hind leg, dig in our heels and pull with everything we've got.

125. The Physician's Duties:
    - Diagnose
    - Treat
    - Relieve suffering
    - Reassure
    - Educate
    - Prevent illness

126. When you pull out the big guns remember big guns leave big holes.

127. White coat and stethoscope win you no respect. If you wanted to be treated like a doctor, act like one.

128. No doctor can heal a patient who does not wish to get well.

129. Staph nests in plastic.

130. At times you'll have to climb down into the grave to bring your patient back to the living. Bring a ladder.

131. A patient discharged still suffering from their chief complaint is a boomerang thrown hard.

132. Things not written in the chart never happened.

133. Almost nothing in medicine is "always" or "never." Almost everything is "usually," "sometimes," "often," and "rarely."

134. Get on the field. Put yourself in the game. Try to win despite bad odds. You might get dirty. You might get bloody. You will lose some. Do it anyway. Do it again.

135. Choose your words carefully. Your patients will repeat them back to you word-for-word years later.

136. Sometimes it feels like losing when a patient dies.
    - I don't like losing.
    - I wouldn't want a doctor who didn't like winning.

137. The Universal Format for a Medical Plan:
    - Name the problem
    - List possible diagnoses
    - List tests to sort them out
    - List the treatments

138. Sometimes it feels like everyone in the hospital is trying to prevent you from taking care of the next patient. Build your team from them.

139. They can't nail you in your coffin while you're walking. Keep walking and you'll live forever.

140. You probably aren't as good as you think you are. You probably aren't as bad as you think you are, either.

141. If the patient is 93 and takes no medicines, try not to ruin it.

142. Knowing how sick your patient is: Arithmetic. Anticipating how sick you patient is going to be: Calculus.

143. Turn all difficult clinical problems into multiple-choice questions. That's why we've been giving you multiple-choice questions since you were 6!

144. The fastest ways to spoil the single doctor's carefree and jolly professional life in the hospital is to date within its walls.

145. There is someone who wanted to be a doctor more than you. Live your dream and theirs too.

146. The Three Essential Steps:
    1. Diagnose and treat the disease
    2. Diagnose and treat the complications of the treatment
    3. Catch your errors as they occur

147.   There are two kinds of people:
       1) Help! This patient needs a doctor!
       2) I am this patient's doctor.

148.   60% of medicine is knowing what is happening.
       40% is predicting what will happen next.

149.   If you can't explain your decisions, you don't
       understand them.

150.   All blood exists in a tenuous balance between
       pouring out onto the floor and clotting solid in
       the vein.

151.   Three things every old person wishes they had
       started with more of:
       1. cartilage
       2. neurons
       3. continence

152.   Guaranteed recipe for success:
       a) Find someone who has succeeded
       b) Befriend them
       c) Imitate them

153. You can't fight dogma with dogma. Fight dogma with evidence.

154. Medicine is a simple set of a few million rules, some of which contradict each other. Good medicine is proper application of rule-breaking.

155. A Short List of Truths:
   - All fevers are intermittent.
   - All delirium waxes and wanes.
   - All blood pressures are variable.
   - All automated platelet counts are estimates.

156. Most human illnesses are cause by:
   - The patient's own body
   - A mean microbe
   - A guy with a gun
   - Sex

The Decision to Become a Physician

157.   If you want to be a doctor, I would encourage
        you. There is no better job in the world.

158.   There have always been, and will always be,
        physicians. The respect they engender will vary
        over time but never vanish.

159.   Try not to forget why you chose this profession.
        You could have been a banker if you preferred.
        You could still be one if you like.

160.   What makes a doctor good is brains, judgment
        and kindness. What makes a one great is
        willingness to see the illness from the patient's
        view.

161.   While there are easier ways to make a living than
        being a doctor, there are not better ways—it's a
        calling to an ancient purpose.

162. A doctor is a person who runs towards screaming and blood while others run away.

163. Competency is not sufficient, you must be caring. Caring is not sufficient, you must be competent.

164. If you do not like clinical medicine, get out of it today. —Clifton K. Meador, MD

165. The joy of becoming a doctor is only slightly tempered by the gradual realization that you've lost the freedom to be mediocre.

166. Some axioms are repeats. Like this one was! When you find one, email me at medicalaxioms@gmail.com!

167. You may not have been born compassionate, caring or smart enough. Not a problem. Great doctors are not born. It's something you become.

168. Great doctors are not defined by the height of their successes but by the shallowness of their failures. Experience will show you that "Do no harm" is an unrealistic expectation. Instead, minimize harm.

169. There are moments when good enough won't do and you'll have to be perfect. They are rare. G slow and careful and double-check your work. You can do it!

170. Once you have decided you were put on this earth to heal the sick, dedicate your life to that end. Do whatever is necessary to maintain your faith in that purpose.

171. If not you, then who will stand between this patient and the grave?

172. Without kindness you are a mechanic. Without technical skill you could be a minister. With both, you may be a physician.

173. You'll never be paid for the minutes of kindness you show a patient on their worst day. You won't have lost a penny, either.

174. Against forces that attempt to derail you, there is no better defense than attention to your professional relationship with your patients.

175. Few patients should die in the hospital with only one doctor.

176. A successful career as a doctor depends upon:
     a) Making sure there is no other career you could do better and
     b) Doing it as it should be done.

177. A valiant effort is often appreciated even when it fails. Nobody appreciates hard work when you make it look easy.

178. Good medicine is a selfless act.

Habit and Character

180. The best time to make a good first impression is
      when you first meet.

181. I always announce myself as I enter the room
      "Dr. Reid here!" and a second time as I depart
      "Dr. Reid says goodbye!" The extroduction is
      more important than the introduction.

182. The case that is baffling to you is simple for your
      colleague and visa versa. Together, we succeed.

183. Only patients truly know who the good doctors
      are.

184. It is more difficult to be an honorable man for a
      week than to be a hero for fifteen minutes. —
      Jules Renard, 1907

185. I've learned most of my bedside manner from my
      dog.

186. Ability exceeding Confidence is humble.
Confidence exceeding Ability is deadly.

187. When delivering bad news, where you choose to sit in the hospital room is nearly as important as what you have to say.

188. Call your failures "failures" without guilt or shame. Critique your worst decisions as if they were made by someone else and you may improve.

189. Instead of saying, "Your CT PE was negative," say, "Good news! We looked for a blood clot in your lungs and we don't see one. What a relief!!"

190. When we say "practice of medicine," we mean it like a concert pianist means it. Not learning how but keeping and honing skills through regular repetition.

191. We don't defeat Death—we only teach him patience.

192. Try not to give the impression that you don't care. Easier by caring. Harder by acting.

193. One of the joys of medicine is meeting sweet little old ladies who can make you blush when they swear like drunken sailors.

194. A good doctor is like a buoy in the ocean—can be turned over by a big wave but flips back upright again in a moment without complaint or apology.

195. Some doctors see nice patients all day while others see horrible ones. The clay does not shape the potter.

196. When you do things for the right reason you are invincible. Ignore the fact that this is not always true.

197. Unused preparation is preferable to unprepared catastrophe.

198. People are happy to see their dog because their dog is always happy to see them. A good doctor is like this.

199. If there's one person in the world who doesn't think she's god, it's the doctor praying she can keep her sickest patient alive through the night.

200. See the healthy person hiding inside the sick one like Michelangelo saw David hiding in a block of marble.

201. If you look for trouble, you'll find it. If you don't look for trouble, it will find you.

202. The practice of medicine requires acting. Your primary role is The Caring Doctor Who has Nothing but Time.

203. You need not be born brilliant. Imitate brilliance.

204. Be the doctor you wish to have in the world.

205. Learn from experience or remain forever a novice.

206. You will never be good enough to speak ill of another doctor in front of a patient.

207. Find a way to bring the greatest benefit to your patients while leaving yourself with the minimum irritation, frustration, and resentment.

208. People die every day for no good reason. Nobody's allowed to do that while I'm looking after them.

209. You may be your patient's only advocate.

210. You learn to apologize the same way you learn everything—practice. Practice often and you will gain mastery.

211. If you do not feel sympathy and compassion, just act it. Keep acting it and you'll start feeling it.

212. Be your own best role model: Do what you think the best person would do in this situation. Inspire yourself!

213. Have fun with the fun patients. Don't have fun with despairing patients. Don't despair with despairing patients.

214. Electronic Health Record: An expensive contraption that makes the ancient practice of ministering to the sick into a video game.

215. I don't provide different care for prisoners. Or foreigners, addicts, millionaires, saints, or "VIPs." Usual practice is always best practice.

216. Old doctors are seldom as good as they think they are. Confidence wears off slower than skill.

217. Doctors are remembered for their good dispositions and bad decisions.

218. Good medicine is done fast. The best medicine is done good and fast.

219. Too much attention can make you inattentive. Sometimes be like a hungry tiger stalking its prey. Other times like a kitten chasing its tail.

220. Remember your purpose: You were put on Earth to heal the sick.

221.   Be stern or gentle as the situation dictates.

222.   You will fail because you are human. When you do, admit your mistake and join your place in humanity. Make an adjustment and get back to work immediately.

223.   All day long treat the sick like usual. At least once a day, perform a good deed.

224.   The proper response to receiving any information about a hospitalized patient from any source no matter how incorrect or useless is, "Thanks for letting me know!"

225.   The closer you get to perfection the more blind you become to your own mistakes.

226.   Some things "are" while others "seem," "suggest" or "appear." Know the difference between facts and hypotheses.

227.   The good doctor anticipates the next step in a hospitalization like a good waiter takes your salad plate or brings the dessert menu: Right on time.

228. It's okay to be different doctors for different patients. Adjust your character and disposition as conditions warrant. Be authentic in your effectiveness.

229. By the last day of a stretch of days you are about 20% worse than usual. Give an extra 20% to make up for it. For interns, this means April, May and June.

230. Patients love to watch you work—look things up, discuss with nurses and colleagues, make phone calls, review labs & x-rays. They want to see you earn your pay.

231. Seasoned physicians simultaneously work faster and take more time with their patients than rookies. It's a skill that cannot be taught. Only learned.

232. Most sick people want to know 2 things:
   - You are on their side
   - You will fight to the death

233. No patient should have a plastic tube inserted in their body without fair warning.

234. Never take medical advice from people who aren't in medicine. Unless it's your mom. Even then, ask for a reference.

235. Farmers and doctors know every hour before 8am is worth two at the end of the day.

236. Medical errors, mistakes, and near misses should only be discussed with colleagues face-to-face in person. Never in the chart.

237. All calls for routine consultations on patients admitted the night before should be made before noon today. It's just good manners.

238. Important orders should be discussed with the patient's nurse before they are written. "I am about to put in an order for ___."

239. As they grow old, doctors have a tendency to grow sullen, solitary and self-righteous. To prevent this, never refuse an invitation to join another person to walk, talk, eat or meet! Go out in public. Make new friends. Stay connected!

240. Doctors don't get burned out because they work too hard. They get burned out because they choose to work too hard on stupid stuff.

241. It is not enough to be good. Aspire to be great. The patient lying in their hospital bed rarely has another option.

242. Usual care is optimal care. Any deviations from usual care are sub-optimal. [Don't think I don't know this is a repeat!]

243. The patient wants you to bring about half of your humanity to work with you—all that is hopeful, kind, attentive, gentle & jolly. Leave the rest at home.

244. In your career, you can choose to develop your defensiveness or your humility. One protects your ego; the other contributes to your ability.

245. Lack of an orderly system to keep track of details is responsible for more medical errors than lack of brilliance.

246. Deplasticate! Every day, identify all plastic tubing in the patient and either remove it or make a plan to, soon.

247. The last patient you want to see today is often the first one you should visit.

248. You aren't as good at the end of the shift, the end of the day, and the end of the week. By the time you get there, you can't tell.

249. Before I leave the room, have a standard script. Something like:
    - ✓ I think I can help you
    - ✓ We will do what we can
    - ✓ I am here to help
    - ✓ I believe I can make you better
    - ✓ Whichever one you choose, make sure it's not a lie!

250. There is no better company for the weary physician than her dog.

251.   A good doctor is a better listener than a talker, but don't forget patients love to tell friends and family what you're like. Especially if you're like a human.

252.   When you hear Danskos running, get ready to run.

253.   A physician can either hone their defensiveness or their humility. One protects the dullness of ego; the other sharpens the blade of skill.

254.   Someone will come to you seeking help today. Put aside your worries, fears and frustrations. Do what you can to help.

255.   Without kindness you are a mechanic. Without technical skill you could be a minister. With both, you may be a physician. This is a repeat.

256.   In the hospital, as in life, neither sponsor nor suffer gossip.

257. Steps to Greatness:
    1. Define great.
    2. Decide to be great.
    3. Find great people around you and ask them, "How did you get here?"
    4. Imitate great until you get there.

258. No patient ever said, "My doctor spent too much time with me and gave me too much information."

259. Axes are to chop wood and shovels are to dig. The doctor is a tool to diagnose, treat, and relieve suffering.

260. Be sure there is no lie when you tell the sick man, "I am working hard to get you well."

261. *~Always Pretty Good~* is preferable to *~Usually Wonderful and Occasionally Abysmal~*.

262. Careful study of a lifetime of little failures will lead to a lifetime of great successes.

263. As you walk into the patient's room, introduce yourself then fix anything that immediately needs fixing: The beeping IV pump, untangle the O2 tubing, fetch a pitcher of water, etc. Now you are ready to talk.

264. Talking to a patient with the TV on in the room is like proposing to your girlfriend at the mall.

265. A scared doctor is of no use to a scared patient.

266. It's okay to look up labs, read journal articles, and write your note in the patient's room. Like your kids and your dog, your patients would rather *be-with-you-not-talking* than *not-be-with-you*.

267. Never make a clinical decision without first deciding what you'll do if you are wrong.

268. Take ownership. Take responsibility. The sick person in front of you remains your patient until someone else takes over.

269. Leaving a patient's room angry is accepting an unnecessary burden.

270. Telling a patient you'll be back after rounds to discuss the new diagnosis of cancer is like giving the girl a ring before work and telling her you'll propose later when you get home from the gym.

271. I tell my patients, "I'm your doctor and I'm here to fix problems." It's a statement of duty, not a promise of outcome.

272. The practice of medicine at top speed and peak performance produces few memories: It's a place of flow somewhere between trance and meditation.

273. If you didn't have fun being a doctor this week it's because you are doing it wrong. Join us on Twitter @medicalaxioms!

274. Each medical interaction is a deal: You are making an agreement to exchange personal information and trust for a chance at diagnosis and treatment.

275. When I leave a patient's room, I say "I will do my best to get you better!" It's a promise I can keep. It generates hope.

Reputation

276. The reputation of our profession hangs on your personal reputation.

277. No matter how talented you are, you are a little better if you're not a jerk.

278. The only true judge of a doctor's quality is a patient who has been seen by her.

279. A great doctor is loved by her patients and revered by her colleagues. Achieving either is difficult. Both will take a lifetime of effort.

280. If you want to earn respect in the hospital, respect your patients at all times and above all else. When nurses and fellow physicians come to you for their care, you will know you are respected.

281. If all else fails, just act like a good doctor in an old movie.

282. Better to practice good medicine from a few years ago than bad medicine.

283. CPR works poorly in the hospital but better than in the mortuary.

284. Nobody wants their doctor to be: Rushed, busy, aloof, angry, sad, nervous, or scared. Humble and uncertain are okay.

285. Your patients will remember the things you say for the rest of their lives. Try not to say anything stupid.

286. "Above all things be strictly temperate." — William Osler, MD

Attitude

287.   'Tis a privilege to be a doctor.

288.   The way to feel capable, optimistic and unstoppable is to act capable, optimistic and unstoppable. Keep doing it until you feel it.

289.   Thank your patients for entrusting their care to you.

290.   When it gets busy, quit talking. Start fixing.

291.   Daily Challenge: Fulfill the promise of the personal statement you wrote on your medical school application.

292.   Success in clinical practice requires estimating how much effort to put into different problems: Little for little, big for big.

293. Never take career advice from someone who hates their job.

294. Why is medicine such a wonderful job? Caring for others makes your own problems vanish.

295. Many doctors are unsatisfied at work. It's not because the job is unsatisfying. It's what they chose to do at the job.

296. A successful career as a doctor depends upon: a) Making sure there is nothing else you could do better and b) Doing it as it should be done. Yes I know that c) This is a repeat.

297. Fastest Road to Burnout: Do non-doctor tasks that you hate.

298. While you cannot always fix everything, there is always something you can do to help.

299. No sick person wants to see Dr. Frowny Face. The will to get well is sponsored by hope and enthusiasm.

300. There is a magical hour when hospital graham crackers and peanut butter tastes like Thanksgiving dinner at your mama's house.

301. Never miss a patient's birthday in the hospital.

302. Hospital: The only place in the world where church and chemistry lab are 20 steps apart.

303. You'll learn more about improving your practice from angry patients than happy ones.

304. See the sickest patient first. Also, never be afraid to repeat yourself like I do with this axiom.

305. All VA patient rooms smell vaguely of cigarettes and maple syrup.

306. The only two people who should ever routinely share a hospital bed are a mom and a newborn.

307. Patients who are having romantic relations in their hospital room are ready for discharge.

308. If there is a "closed intensive care unit," floor doctors decide which patients should go to the ICU and ICU doctors decide which patients go to the floor. This is ancient tradition.

309. Learn how to fetch a blanket and fill the water pitcher.

310. Every job in the hospital is easier criticized than done. Especially yours.

311. I asked an old lady patient if she had any advice regarding sex. She said, "Have more when you are young. You can read books later."

312. Message to Patients: You'll get better medical care if you are nice to the people caring for you.

313. Some doctors in the hospital secrete a pheromone that attracts the vacuum cleaner to them wherever they go.

314. The best way to get a patient out of bed and walking is tell him you'll stop his heparin shots if he does.

315. Hypothesis: Patients in double rooms have lower mortality than private rooms. A roommate can be better supervision than a telemetry monitor.

316. Irrespective of diagnosis, 99% of patients admitted after 10pm would like a turkey sandwich.

317. Percent of healthcare worker who make healthy eating choices between 2am and 5am: 0.2%.

318. If you have to put a needle in someone, do it quick.

319. You can kill a man by confining him to bed for a week.

320. You'll spend so much time in the hospital, it will start to feel like home. It isn't.

321. Placement of an NG tube is a routine bedside procedure when performed on someone else.

322. At times you must clean your inpatient service like Hercules cleaned the king's stables.

323. The Lord helps those who help themselves, but not at the Pyxis.

324. Life in the hospital is easier if you make sure everyone owes you a favor.

325. Once you have spent untold hours, nights, weekends and holidays in the hospital, the middle of a normal weekday feels like the easiest thing you have ever done.

326. ACLS class is like voting—a moment of equality among all healthcare providers in the practice of civic duty.

327. As in chess, there are times in medicine when the best next move involves a sacrifice.

328. Hospitals are commonly mistaken for:
     1) A hotel
     2) A restaurant
     3) A travel agency
     4) Their mom's house

329. For doctors, getting a new hospital computer system is like being forced to change religions.

330. The best medical decisions are not made too slow or too fast. The ideal pace feels a little faster than you might like.

331. Your patient has often waited 23 hours and 55 minutes to see you again. Catch up on the news by asking, "What's happened since I saw you last?"

Nurses and Nursing

333.   Dismiss the suggestion of a good nurse once and you may lose a valuable stream of information forever.

334.   Every nurse can tell you quick and accurate if a patient in a ward bed should be in the ICU and visa versa.

335.   Never ignore an experienced nurse who is telling you that a patient is dying.

336.   At the 3rd call...
- from any nurse,
- about anything,
- on any patient,
- at any time,
- ... go to the room and see the patient with your own eyes.

337.   The bed sucks strength from the sick.

338. Befriend all nurses and romance none.

339. The best way to stop diarrhea is to order stool to be collected and sent to the lab. —Rachel Cruz, RN

340. Once a nurse decides a patient is up to no good, his reputation will not recover.

341. Thank nurses for all the calls they don't make to you every night.

342. When you tell a new nurse to remove a fentanyl patch, remind him to wear gloves.

History: *Stop talking. Let the patient tell you what is wrong with them.*

344.   Most diagnoses are made from the history.

345.   Create an awkward silence. Your patient will step into it and tell their story.

346.   Some patients can tell you exactly what wrong with them. Others can't. You can't tell them apart.

347.   Learning to take a history is simply learning to apply an orderly structure to your natural curiosity.

348.   When a patient has multiple symptoms, the most important question is "Which came first?"

349.   Often neglected but important history question: What made you finally decide to seek care?

350. Of simultaneous pain in two places, the lesser is obliterated by the greater. —Hippocrates

351. Patients don't deny [symptom]. They simply do not have [symptom].

352. When you go back to take a history on a patient who has seen many doctors, the most important question is: What did you notice first?

353. Criminals deny and complainers complain. Patients *have* symptoms or habits or they *do not have them*.

354. When the patient lives with the daughter and she says he doesn't seem right, something is not right.

355. Hidden in the words of almost every patient's chief complaint is a simple request: "Please help me."

356. The first thing lost as the patient enters the hospital is the chief complaint. You can find it again by asking: What was the first thing you noticed? What made you decide to come to the hospital?

357. The Essential Elements of the History:
- The first symptom
- The order symptoms occurred
- The reason the patient finally sought care

358. You will never know:
✓ Who is hurting
✓ Who is lying
✓ When you think you can tell, you know something: You suffer a delusion.

359. If you keep quiet, the patient will usually tell you what is wrong with them.

360. There is no illness more serious than the one that causes the dry cleaning lady to close up her own shop and come to the hospital.

361. You'll never convince a patient they do not have their symptoms.

362. In medicine, better occasionally deceived than always doubting.

363. I get the same excitement when I sit down to take a history that I get when the curtains open and a play begins in the theater. I love to hear a story!

364. When 3 or more physicians are involved in a case the majority is often correct. Not always.

365. It is not always the most interesting job in the world, but from time to time you will hear the most interesting stories.

366. The question "What are your symptoms?" is a very different question than "Why are you here?"

367. Yesterday's history is like day old bread. Maybe a little stale but it might be the best thing you get for a long time.

368.   Most valuable parts of the physical exam:
    1. Vital signs
    2. General appearance
    3. Orientation questions

369.   Respect all objective findings—things measured with instruments and recorded as numbers. They cannot be denied.

370.   More people die from low blood pressures than high. Faster too.

371.   If a patient's normal BP is 180/120, he's half dead at 90/60.

372.   The most important physical finding is not something you see. It's something you feel in your own guts.

373.   The room, including the people and stuff in it, is part of the physical examination.

374. Never leave the socks on a hospitalized patient. There may be something hiding in there that wants to kill them. Don't forget to put them back on when you are done.

375. Sport Ball Sizes in Medicine for tumors, masses and abscesses: BB, marble, ping pong ball, golf ball, racquetball, tennis ball, softball, football, basketball, beach ball.

376. Food Sizes in Medicine: Poppy seed, peppercorn, pea, grape, egg, orange, grapefruit, cantaloupe, pumpkin, watermelon.

377. If we have ever met, I have examined your nails. I'm never not looking for clubbing.

378. The JVP is one of the most useful physical findings in medicine. Unless you can't see it in which case it is useless.

Laboratory Tests and Radiology

380.   The most sensitive diagnostic test is a little nerve in the center of you chest. When it feels scared, somebody might be getting ready to die.

381.   No single *isolated* blood test is less informative than the abnormal white blood cell count between 4,000 and 20,000.

382.   Some of our tools are dangerous. Don't fear them. Like a carpenter, master their safe use.

383.   The definition of an unnecessary test is one where neither a positive result nor a negative result will change management.

384.   If you don't intend to look at the result, don't order the test. If you won't be the one to see the result of the test, think carefully before ordering.

385.   All unnecessary tests are obviously worthless once you know the result.

386. Objective findings are indelible, irrefutable, invaluable, and easy to display as exhibits at trial.

387. A negative test result can be more valuable than a positive one.

388. Daily labs do not contribute much to anemia: At 5cc per tube x 3 tubes a day (red, purple, blue), it takes 30 days to steal a unit (450cc = HCT-3%, or Hgb-1gm/dL) of blood from a patient.

389. The white blood cell count in the blood goes up and down. Sometimes it is something and sometimes it is nothing.

390. Objective measures (things with numbers) have three essential qualities: 1) Their current value, 2) Their trajectory, 3) Their acceleration.

391. When we get a lab value that we don't like, we repeat it. If we like the 2nd number better than the 1st, we call the first one a lab error. This is usually but not always true.

392. There are two important things to know about every lab test:
- What is the result today?
- Which direction is the result moving and how fast?

393. You will never order so many CT scans for aortic dissection as during the first month after you miss one.

394. Few diagnostic tests cost more than another day in the hospital.

395. Urine was invented to find liars who "are not sexually active" and "never use illicit drugs." And to surprise women who "can't possibly be pregnant."

396. A radiology test feels like an objective test. The fact that it requires the interpretation of a radiologist makes it subjective.

Diagnosis

397. Never wait for an answer that should be found immediately.

398. Don't ask a question if you don't need to know the answer.

399. The only diagnoses that can be made with 100% certainty are traumatic amputation and death. Death is harder than you think.

400. It is not to be imagined that he should know the remedies of diseases who knows not their original causes. —Celsus

401. The experienced physician should be able to judge with confidence how confident they are of every judgment they make. Rookies have no clue and that's to be expected.

402. Never be afraid to abandon your most confident diagnosis when presented with compelling evidence you are wrong.

403. Good rules work usually. No rules work universally.

404. Making a diagnosis changes management by allowing you to stop looking for a diagnosis.

405. No diagnosis is wrong until a superior diagnosis is made.

406. A working diagnosis should never be abandoned—only replaced by a better one.

407. If you can't decide what to do next, make a list of all the things you could do. Pick the best one. (Now you know why we have given you millions of multiple question tests during your medical education)

408. If it walks like a duck and quacks like a duck, it's a duck. Or a platypus with a cough.

409.   If you can't find a diagnosis, it's either hiding high up yonder in that tree or right under your shoe.

410.   Not ordering tests prevents you from making diagnoses but it doesn't prevent patients from dying from them.

411.   Always start your differential diagnosis with real diseases that kill people. End with stupid stuff that does nothing. After that, faking and drug-seeking.

412.   Nothing saves money like a diagnosis.

413.   You'll make your best medical decisions out loud, in the patient's room, in real time, with the help of patient, nurse and family.

414.   "It's all in your head" is less convincing to the worried patient seeking help than "I have considered and searched for the likely life-threatening causes of your symptoms and find no sign of any of them."

415.   Know what is possible. Even when it is unlikely.

416. Don't waste time ruling out a bunch of stuff the patient doesn't have. Just figure out what she does.

417. The more common a disease, the more common its mimics.

418. The fact that a diagnosis is rendered by a specialist does not guarantee that the diagnosis is correct.

419. You can put "faking" on every differential diagnosis you make if it's important to you. Just put it dead last.

420. It's usually possible to name a disease that explains all the relevant findings that is utterly wrong. For example, "viral syndrome."

421. Discard your best theory without fanfare or remorse when it is proven wrong. Move logically to the next most likely item on your differential diagnosis.

422. The Humbling Cycle of Medical Practice:
   - You will be wrong.
   - You will hear about it.
   - You will be ashamed.
   - You will discover your error and learn to avoid it
   - You will be a better doctor afterwards.

423. Don't worry about being right all the time. Do your best to avoid being wrong.

424. A list of possibilities is more likely partially correct than a single diagnosis.

425. The first thing we teach you in med school is to recognize the familiar. It'll take years of practice to learn to recognize the unfamiliar.

426. The differential diagnosis with only one item is a logical failure. Once ruled out, you are back to having no idea what your patient has.

427. The two things your patient has that most people don't have are trunk and tail of the same elephant.

428. The decision to seek a diagnosis with further testing instead of simply reassuring the patient that nothing is wrong comes from the stomach, not the brain.

429. Only god and the pathologist know for certain what is wrong when the patient presents. The pathologist may need additional stains. The rest of us must rely on clues and intuition.

430. Let the patient and their family add to your differential diagnosis, never subtract from it.

431. If it could be this disease or that one, and both are deadly, treat both while you figure it out.

432. The nose is the most neglected diagnostic tool.

433. If there is a tool applying objective criteria to make a diagnosis (e.g. Duke Criteria for bacterial endocarditis), use it.

434. A diagnosis is like a pair of new shoes: Try it on and wear it around for a bit before you decide if it fits.

435. When you hear hoof beats and see an elephant, it's an elephant.

436. The correct diagnosis may be only part of what's wrong.

437. Guard against the Ancient Truth: When the doctor cannot find disease, the patient becomes a liar.

438. Your first intuitive guess is often right. Abandon intuition without remorse when it's proven wrong.

439. Unrelated coincidences are uncommon.
      ➢ Find the two things your patient has that nearly no one else has.
      ➢ Find a disease that explains both.

440. It's difficult to diagnose a disease you have never seen before, even when it's staring you right in the face.

441. When you hear hoofbeats behind you, don't expect to see a zebra. —Theodore E. Woodward

442. When you are lost:
- Don't lose your head
- Be systematic
- Name the possibilities
- Make a plan for sorting them
- Ask for help

443. Even a slow illness can beat you with a big head start.

444. The two most common cognitive errors in diagnosis:
- ✓ Never thought of it and
- ✓ Thought of it but was sure he didn't have it.

445. It's hard to make a diagnosis you can't name.

446. The Coin Method to decide between two equally likely diagnoses:
   a) Assign one diagnosis heads and the other tails
   b) Flip the coin and look at it
   c) Announce the diagnosis made by the coin
   d) Then say, "Never let a stupid coin make a complex medical decision!"
   e) Pick the correct diagnosis

447. A physician who has never seen your patient can add to your differential diagnosis. Don't let them subtract from it.

448. As in taking a test, in clinical situations your first guess is usually the best. Trust your gut.

449. The best surprise is "I can't believe this test is negative!" Much preferable to reading autopsy report and thinking, "Wow she really had it..."

450. As a patient you are better off with a doctor who says, "I don't know" than a doctor who has a quick answer for everything.

451. Patients admitted with chest pain often have fascinating stories that nobody ever hears.

452. No matter how good you get, sometimes you'll miss one. Remember:
    - Little better than big
    - Early better than late
    - Live better than dead

453. Test not done are not negative. Pending results are not negative.

454. Your patient in the cemetery doesn't want to hear the next test you would have ordered.

455. When in doubt, do something to lessen it.

456. Never let an inexpensive, non-invasive diagnostic test stand between you and a life-threatening diagnosis.

457. There are two presentations that do not require a differential diagnosis: 1) Traumatic amputation. 2) Visible baby head.

458. I have heard more than one doctor tell this woeful tale: I thought of it, but did not test for it. The patient had it, and died from it.

459. An unusual presentation of common disease is more likely than a common presentation of an unusual disease. Someone famous said this.

460. No one ever died of a chest x-ray. People have died from a missed pneumonia, pleural effusion, aortic dissection, and pericardial effusion

461. Nature pays no heed to your certainty that the patient does not have a diagnosis.

462. Solving difficult cases is like surviving lost in the woods.
    1) Stay alive
    2) Stop walking—don't get any more lost than you already are
    3) Maintain faith you will prevail
    4) If available, assemble a team before you proceed

463. Trust your gut. When you feel angry or scared there is dissonance. This discomfort is valuable information. Find the part that does not fit.

464. The diagnosis most missed was never considered.

465. It's better to find the diagnosis than to be found by the doctor who found it.

466.   Rather practice a few years behind than miss a
         diagnosis that Galen could have made.

467.   Even for the "easy" and "obvious" cases,
         maintain a short differential diagnosis. Cellulitis
         could be Sweet's; COPD exacerbation could be a
         PE; sepsis could be adrenal insufficiency...

468.   Bad doctors correctly make difficult diagnoses.
         Good doctors miss easy ones. Thus the
         distinction between them is unclear.

469.   In the end, diagnosis is 50% seeing what is there,
         40% predicting the future, and 10% coin flip.

470.   In the elderly, Occam's razor is a Swiss Army
         knife.

471.   Faced with conflicting evidence, objective
         findings almost always outweigh subjective.

472.   Ask about chest pain and you will hear about
         chest pain. You won't always hear why the
         patient came to the hospital.

473. Remain a little skeptical of any diagnosis made by someone else. Expect them to do the same to you.

474. You will be remembered forever by a few people for a few of the diagnoses you miss.

475. When you are right, thank your gods you are right. When you are wrong, thank your gods if nobody dies before you find it.

476. There are no new medical illnesses; only old ways to be tricked and trapped by them.

477. Often without awareness, you make this important decision many times a day:
    - Taking the concern seriously and embarking on a diagnostic adventure or
    - Dismissing it as nothing.

478. The most accurate diagnostic test is the autopsy. It's pretty invasive.

479.   Tests don't order themselves. The doctor
        ordering the test makes the diagnosis, not the
        test.

Treatment

481. You don't understand a disease until you learn the complications of its treatment.

482. All effective drugs have side effects. Any drug with no side effects has no effect.

483. Like seeds in a farmer's field, medicines need time to sprout and grow.
    - ☐ Usually ~5 half-lives
    - ☐ Hint: most drugs are dosed by their half-life

484. The most effective medicines are ones the patient is willing to take.

485. It's easier to give a second small dose of medicine than to take back half a large dose.

486. A prescription is not a commandment. It is a prayer.

487.   The two most effective medicines for chronic pain are exercise and a job.

488.   A slightly outdated treatment is better than a diagnosis as wrong today as 100 years ago.

489.   When prescribing a new medicine, say, "This is very strong medicine!" This gets you a little placebo effect to go with your effect.

490.   Like a carpenter, a good doctor knows how to safely use every tool in the box. Even the ones seldom used.

491.   If you are giving a very expensive medicine it's okay to say, "This medicine is very expensive." It sometimes makes it work better.

492.   The most under-prescribed medicine is a 30 minute walk outside every day.

493.   Two prescriptions are almost always picked up at the pharmacy:
       1) Proton-pump inhibitors
       2) Opiates

494. Never adjust the dose of a medicine the patient does not take.

495. You'll really wish you had a strong indication for a drug when a life-threatening complication develops.

496. If the patient's mouth works, always use the mouth. Otherwise, you can use a vein.

497. Most patients are prescribed more medicines than they need. Most also take fewer than prescribed.

498. Ignoring a little of the doctor's advice is a normal expression of free will.

499. 95% of patients sitting on the edge of the bed with clothes and shoes on are ready for discharge.

500. Email me at medicalaxioms@gmail.com & say hi! ☺

501. You can lie about taking your warfarin but I will find out when I draw your blood. We will find out you aren't taking your rivaroxaban together.

502. You'll make
   - good decisions if you treat patients like family.
   - bad decisions if you treat family as patients.

503. Easier to start a medicine than stop one.

504. Blood tests performed after the first transfusion reflect the condition of donor and recipient.

505. One liter of water in the mouth is the same as one liter of water in the vein.* It's conservation of mass. *Exceptions: Cholera, shock, ileus, and others.

506. Some treatment failures are caused by misdiagnosis.

507. As Rome was not built, neither is essential hypertension fixed, in a day.

508. If you are not running a CODE, stand behind the person running it with a book or card and whisper "I am here to help." Whisper each next right step in their ear as they command the room.

509. It takes a wise doctor to know when not to prescribe, and at times the greater skill consists in not applying remedies. —Gracian, b. 1601

510. It is usually an error to treat the side effect of a medication with another medication. Exception: All of oncology.

511. How to Reassure a Patient:
    - Why did you come in again?
    - What is it you were you worried about?
    - I have good news for you! You do not have that!!

512. Boomerang (n.): A patient discharged home still suffering from the same complaint they came in with.

513. Some beautiful treatment plans that were very difficult to create fall apart immediately because they did not consider the person for whom they were built.

514. The Evil Demons love to find an IV you aren't using anymore so they can stuff Staph in it.

515. The most difficult treatment to deliver is reassurance. Many physicians never master its use.

516. You can't remake yesterday's decisions.
    - Take ownership of them.
    - Learn where they failed.
    - Make better decisions today.

517. Well-made plans that don't succeed outside the hospital are not well-made.

518. There is no surer measure of patient adherence than an INR of 2.5 in a patient who is prescribed warfarin. Except maybe a patient with correctly diagnosed type one diabetes and an A1C of 6.5.

519. Better a firefighter who is afraid of fire than one who is afraid of water.

520. When uncertain, first make a list of what can be done. Now decide what should be done.

521. The answer may not be in any textbook or paper. You will have to use your own good judgment and common sense.

522. Sometimes it's not the chief complaint that causes the 10-day hospital stay. It's the intractable nausea and vomiting.

523. Preparing a patient for discharge is like stocking a ship for a voyage at sea.

524. Pills can be prescribed, filled, picked up and taken home. Their effectiveness is found in the swallowing.

525. The most accurate test for determining the appropriateness of discharge is asking the patient if they are ready to go home.

526. The best time to think about malnutrition in the hospitalized patient is 3 months ago.

The Relief of Suffering

527. God made human beings in pain and the opium poppy. God gave you good judgment to decide when to bring them together.

528. Nothing hurts like pain.

529. "My own professional and personal experience has shown me that morphine is the gift of God..." —Francis Peabody, MD, 1927

530. If the dying patient wants to eat, let them eat.

531. Nobody ever asks for a prescription for opiates while they are laughing. Always keep them laughing while you walk out of the room.

532. You know a patient is hurting when they hold your wrists and stare unblinking in your eyes while you examine them.

533. There is no pain meter on the human body. The only way to know how much someone is hurting is to ask them.

534. Acutely, opiates relieve pain. Chronic use of opiates can make ordinary life unbearably painful.

535. You can't convince someone they are not in pain.

536. Most common lies told in the hospital:
    ☐ This won't hurt a bit.
    ☐ You are going to feel a little pinch.
    ☐ This may sting a bit.
    ☐ You may feel a little burn.

537. Even while you determine the cause of acute pain, it is often reasonable to relieve it.

538. You do not have the magic power to know which patients are hurting.

539. Best time to discuss end-of-life issues with patients:
- ☐ After they get sick
- ☐ Before they are dead

540. When all else fails, relieve suffering. Also, don't wait until all else fails.

541. In the healthy young person, opiate overdose will manifest as sleepy before hypoxia. Old people, those with COPD and others can stop breathing while they look wide awake.

542. The two-step key to happiness:
1. Don't tell patients if they are in pain or how much.
2. Don't let patients tell you what medicines to prescribe or how much.

543. Compassion is like a grapevine. It grows best in fresh air and sunshine in the company of other vines.

544. Nothing makes being sick worse than coincident hunger and thirst. If they can tolerate it, you can relieve a lot of suffering with a simple bag of IV fluids.

545. Trying to figure out which patients deserve your sympathy is a) exhausting, b) not part of your professional duty c) not something you are good at. Distribute compassion evenly.

546. In showing compassion for yourself, you practice for your patients. In showing compassion to your patients, you practice for yourself.

Death and Dying

547. When it is time to discuss death, there is no TV, cellphone or pager. It should be done like a marriage proposal—in a quiet room free of distractions.

548. Never deny a dying person a bowl of ice cream.

549. Walk the dying patient to the end of the dock, make sure she is comfortable in the boat, and wave goodbye as she floats away. Then turn around and walk back to shore.

550. The only funeral I can guarantee you won't cry at is your own.

551. Everyone wants to die suddenly except anyone who just died suddenly.

552. Some dying patients see a roomful of angels. Others a room full of demons. Invite angels.

553. Never give a definite opinion as to how long a patient will live; for the only certainty is, that if you do, you will be wrong. —S. Gee

554. Patients who are dying look like:
   a) they are going over the first big hill on a roller coaster or
   b) they couldn't care less.

555. The four words never to say are "I can't help you." When you tell someone they are going to die soon, you suddenly have lots of things you can do for them.

556. It's surprising how many doctors are willing to have an end-of-life discussion with the TV on in the room.

557. If you want you kid to grow up to be a doctor, get them lots of pets. This will get them used to death.

558. All patients who take their medicines exactly as prescribed are liars.

559. It is nearly impossible to have a decent end-of-life discussion without using the word "god," even if you don't have any god, yourself.

560. Some people say that—when it's time—they'd like to die suddenly. I'd like a week. I have a few calls to make and I'd like a dozen oysters and a pint of Graeters.

561. Master the skill of telling patients when you have nothing left to offer. Then unlearn it. You always have something.

562. It is difficult to have an end-of-life discussion with a person the very first day you meet them. It is not impossible.

563. Nobody should die of a curable disease. You don't know it's curable until you know what it is. Thus, all dying patients deserve a diagnosis.

564.   If you don't at least think about crying when your patient cries, go to the morgue. You're dead.

565.   You should always tell your deceased patient's family you worked hard and did your best. They might believe you if you did.

566.   I once asked an 88 year old what his secret was to long life. He said, "I'm scared of dying."

567.   Some doctors know more about a disease than any of their patients. Some patients know more about having their disease than any doctor.

568.   Make a habit of clearly stating what you can and cannot fix. It will benefit your patients and you as well.

569.   The secret of the care of the patient is in caring for the patient. —Francis W. Peabody, MD

570. "I've seen one of these once" sounds better to the patient's ears than "I've never seen this before!" Still, don't lie if you've never seen it.

571. The treatment of a disease may be entirely impersonal, the care of a patient must be completely personal. —Francis W. Peabody, MD

572. Good Words to Use When Talking to Patients: Germs, salts, water, sugar, blood, lung disease from smoking, weak heart, lump, tumor, growth, shadow, hole, pipe, clog, life, death.

573. Respect the patient who tells you he never takes his medicine.

574. When it comes to his own feet, every man is a surgeon.

575. Don't ask a patient what treatment they want. Let them choose from among the treatments that are available.

576. I let myself dislike two patients a year. I save one for December.

577. Every patient is a mirror. Angry patients show you your anger. Appreciative patients show you the kindness you have shown them.

578. A reasonable response to an unreasonable request: "With apologies, that is not a service we offer."

579. Choose your words carefully. You'll forget them in a minute. Your patients will remember them for a lifetime.

580. The best whisky is taken neat without ice or water. Similarly, important medical information should be delivered directly without dilution.

581. Be always kind and seldom wrong. You are seldom remembered for your rightness. You are long-remembered for your kindness and your wrongness.

582. Try these Good Words: "I have listened to your story and examined you carefully. I have found nothing that will hurt or kill you."

583. Never give bad news with bad breath.

584. Women come to the hospital when they feel sick. Men come to the hospital when women think they are sick.

585. Patients start few unhappy stories about a doctor with "She came in here, pulled up a chair, and introduced herself..."

586. A criticism from a patient is like a cockroach—for every one you see there are a thousand more hiding in the wall.

587. It's an unhappy doctor who is disappointed in his patients' behavior. Remind yourself you aren't his mother, his priest or his parole officer.

588. I admire few things more than a sick person who wants to get well to go back to work or get home to take care of their kids.

589. There are some patients who would rather not hear their diagnosis spoken out loud in the room. None are better off if you keep quiet.

590. The art of medicine consists in amusing the patient while nature cures the disease. —Voltaire

591. Ninety percent of the time, an angry patient has a legitimate concern. Ignore the anger and listen for the free information.

592. If you wish to have your words remembered by your patients, make them memorable.

593. Some patients won't remember what you told them 5 minutes ago. Others will quote you verbatim 20 years from now.

594. No doctor is Genie in a lamp. Some wishes cannot be granted.

595. Don't offer options when there are no options.

596. The better you get, the greater the difference in your speed *between* the rooms and *in* the rooms.

597. When you have nothing left to offer, apologize. It's just good manners.

598. I have never had a patient protest when I turn off the TV when I enter the room. I still always ask.

599. We teach you your job is to rule out life-threatening illness. Your patient actually wants you to tell them what's wrong with them.

600. Five words that will correct many difficult patient interactions and misunderstandings: "I am here to help."

601. We tend to dismiss patients' theories about their diagnosis, but a fresh idea, even when incorrect, is a rare and precious commodity.

602. Good manners and compassion are essential but the greatest kindness you can show your patient is competence.

603. Like pulling off a Band-Aid, bad news hurts less delivered quickly, but with a little warning.

604. Words I use: "We have looked carefully for trouble and we find none. I am reassured that your symptoms are not from anything serious."

605. Words I use: "I know the appearance of thousands of diseases that can hurt or kill you and I see none of them."

606. Words I use: "After these tests we know more about your body than I do about my own. Everything we see looks okay."

607. The "difficult patient" who is suddenly easy to get along with can be a pleasant surprise. Or he's about to die.

608.   You'll be made a fool when you ignore the family who says their person doesn't seem right.

609.   When I pick up a patient from a colleague in the hospital, I get to know them by saying, "I'm Dr. Newguy taking over for Dr. Lastguy. Can you tell me what is wrong with you?"

610.   If your day in the hospital sucks, it's usually because someone else's day is sucking more.

611.   Bad News: The solution to an angry patient is often to spend more time in the room with them and their family.

612.   Any patient who comes to the hospital during the Super Bowl has a decent chance of dying.

613.   People often want to be discharged to get home to their dog. Sometimes to get back to work. That's about it.

614. A good doctor acts like they have all the time in the world but finishes your appointment before it was supposed to start.

615. Your patient is never your opponent. You and your patient are playing doubles against Disease and Nature.

616. Before complaining that your patient does not listen to you, ask yourself if you are saying anything worth hearing.

617. If your patients are your problem, you have a problem.

618. The best time to make a good first impression is when you first meet someone.

620.   Doctors were more respected when we had less to offer.

621.   To the love of his profession the physician should add a love of humanity. —Hippocrates

622.   One of the mysteries of modern medicine is how badly some people wish they were doctors and how badly some doctors wish they were something else.

623.   How can it be that the doctor of the early 20th century had less technology, fewer drugs and made more misdiagnoses but was held in higher esteem?

624.   A doctor is like a dairy cow. They will give for a lifetime if you treat them right. Don't try to get it all this week.

625. Great writers love to write. Great painters love to paint. Great doctors love to hear stories and solve problems.

626. The second number they give when you call a VA hospital is suicide prevention. The casualties of war continue long after combat ceases.

627. Unvaccinated children guarantee future vaccine sales.

628. Many people have their hands in the basket as it passes from patient to doctor.

629. Nothing makes your hospital administrator happier than knowing you aren't in it for the money.

630. Keep bashing the medical profession. One day when you get sick, you will have to go to the bank for help. You'll find the Best and Brightest working there.

631. It is a disturbing waste of healthcare dollars to have a doctor do a task that could be done by someone who is paid less.

632. Observation Status: A simple system by which the people holding the money can avoid paying the people who have done the work.

633. It is a normal human response to turn away from sickness, injury, and blood. In this way, doctors are abnormal.

634. The greatest threat to the status of doctors in America is not policy, profit, or legislation. It is the perception that doctors care more about this stuff than their patients.

635. If you are willing to let the sommelier suggest a wine for you dinner, you should be okay letting your doctor suggest a life saving treatment.

636. If you don't like treating prisoners, just think of it as getting them healthy enough so they can serve every last day of their sentence.

637. In towns with an NFL team, the ED is usually empty during the game and very busy afterwards. This is true of the entire U.S. during the Super Bowl.

638. As much as forces try to make medicine a business, the inside of a hospital is no free market. You can't switch surgeons in the middle of the case.

639. Every U.S.-trained MD is the product of a huge government program. Every resident is a giant public investment.

640. Your enemy is not insurance company, colleague, nor patient wanting opiates. Your enemy is disease.

641. If you ever go to a medical meeting, try to remember to take off your name tag when you go out onto the street. Fewer people will ask you for money.

642. Humbly I confess, no matter what foreign language a patient speaks, I respond first in broken Spanglish.

643. Most patients don't drive to an appointment and pay a copay to hear what disease they don't have. Seek a diagnosis.

644. The anti-vaccine movement proposes to distrust science and medicine. What they truly disrespect is the power of Nature and Her diseases.

645. The sad truth is, while I am far from perfect at it, I am far better at doctoring than I am at the rest of life.

646. The wrong place to try to fix America's broken healthcare system is at the patient's bedside.

647. Don't use the next patient you see to try to fix America's healthcare problem.

648. There are harder jobs than being a doctor. I had a cat named Yi who bit through the vet's thumb joint resulting in multiple weeks of IV antibiotics.

649. Your patient might have nothing wrong with them. People have nothing all the time. They're paying you to make sure it isn't something.

650. Physicians do not care for prisoners, criminals, terrorists or victims. We care for human beings. There is no need to pass judgment.

651. Your Primary Duties to Society:
   - Diagnose and treat.
   - Relieve suffering.
   - Prevent illness.

652.   You invite catastrophe when you second-guess your own physician. You will do it anyway.

653.   The sample closet has been the beginning of many clinical misadventures.

654.   The doctor going to the doctor is the actor going to the theater.

655.   Nothing will teach you how to talk about hospice like talking to your mom about hospice.

656.   When you join a case in progress, human nature dictates you begin by assuming everything is wrong and the other doctors are idiots. It isn't and they aren't.

657.   When you have nothing left to give, ask for help. It is always available when you ask for it.

658.   The doctor who has never seen the patient is always smarter than the idiots busting their butts to keep her alive.

659.   When I was a kid, I wanted to be a doctor. Now that I am a doctor, I want to be the doctor I had as a kid. (Jim Phinney, MD of Cincinnati, Ohio)

660.   Medicine is full of introverts who do a decent job of acting like they are extroverts. Most true extroverts wouldn't last a week.

661.   All doctors are gamblers by nature. Good ones make small bets and play the odds.

662.   The better all the other doctors do, the busier the geriatrician gets.

663.   Arm yourself with sufficient scrutiny to judge your decisions as though they had been made by some other doctor—an incompetent one.

Medical Education: *Medical Students. AKA "studs."*

665. Student, you do not study to pass the test. You study to prepare for the day when you are the only thing between the patient and the grave.

666. If you want to be a doctor, you must be willing to work and study while others play and rest.

667. Every doctor is a role model. Either:
    1. Talk, act, and be like me or
    2. Never ever talk, act or be like me

668. Learn from experience or remain forever a novice.

669. The indications for admission should rarely come from the ROS. If it does, rewrite the HPI.

670. Do the things you hate first. And fast.

671. When you meet a new patient remember this: For somewhere between 5 minutes and 50 years, they have been waiting to tell their story to someone who will listen.

672. If you want to be smarter than everyone else you are going to have to work harder than everyone else.

673. The definition of teaching is saying something that cannot be forgotten.

674. Medical Student, talent may have gotten you here but only hard work will get you where you're going.

675. Valid criticism from a capable instructor is a gift.

676. Criticism from people who don't know you that sounds worthless often is.

677. If you don't have anything to do, go in the loneliest patient's room. Sit and talk for an hour. You'll both benefit.

678. On the first day of the rotation, I tell medical students, "I value integrity, hard work, enthusiasm, and brains. In that order."

679. Medical school and residency are easy if you decide beforehand there is no other job for you.

680. The lesson students learn faster than any other is that all patients are liars, cheats, and complainers. Never teach this lesson.

681. Curiosity is the foundation of good history-taking. Follow your curiosity!

682. Your teachers come bearing gifts. Some are pearls, others pebbles. Collect them all. It may take years to tell them apart.

683. We've taught you plenty but if we haven't taught you to advocate for your patients—defend the defenseless—we've taught you nothing.

684. "Half of what we are going to teach you is wrong, and half of it is right. Our problem is that we don't know which half is which." —Charles Sidney Burwell

685. It's good to be smart. Better to be hard working. Indispensable to be willing.

686. If someone has a better system than you, use it.

687. As a general rule, a medical student shouldn't try to tell an old doctor what can happen within the human body.

688. Master bluffing and you'll never learn medicine.

689. Before you can teach a student to love medicine, you must love it.

690. A medical student gets negligible returns on investment of effort before 90% of maximum and big returns after.

691. Why was I born? Why did I study? Why did I work while other people slept, vacationed, and celebrated? Because I have a purpose—to heal the sick.

692. Pay no attention to how much work there is to be done. The only task that can be done is the next one.

693. Medical knowledge is best taken with a spoon not a shovel.

694. In anatomy it is better to have learned and lost than never to have learned at all.

695. How do you work with people you hate? Hating people is a luxury you can't afford in medicine.

696. Few diagnoses instill so much anxiety in a new intern as the first pronouncement of death.

697. Medicine is learned by the bedside and not in the classroom. —William Osler

698.   Anatomy is learned from books and practiced on a cadaver, not the other way around.

699.   You want to be perfect but you can't be perfect. Learn to tolerate being good enough but insist on getting better.

700.   How do human beings survive outside the hospital without daily labs and electrolyte repletion? Dumb luck. 3.5 billion years of dumb luck.

701.   Residents don't get burned out because they work too hard. They get burned out because they choose to focus attention on non-rewarding tasks. Focus on caring for the sick.

702.   Your greatness will never be found in your grades or income. It will be found in your compassion and persistence.

703.   One easy way to high marks on your inpatient clinical rotations is to answer "yes" to any reasonable request for anything related to the care of your patients.

704. For most good, enthusiastic hard-working students, the difference between honors and high pass is the score on the shelf exam. You must study books while working on the wards!

Interns and Residents

706. New interns, bring us your optimism, enthusiasm, and drive. They are the fuels that stoke the fires of medical education!

707. Number of tasks you must complete in a day: Infinity. Number of tasks you can do next: One.

708. The Intern's Prayer: May I learn all the ways my patients can die a little faster than they die from them.

709. The patient you don't want to see at all today, see first.

710. Interns who don't check their check boxes give me hives. Interns that don't have checkboxes give me anaphylaxis.

711. Experience is a good teacher, but she sends in terrific bills. —Minna Antrim

712.   Strive to end each day neither dehydrated nor angry.

713.   A good question to ask every patient: "How will I know when you are better?"

714.   Rookies attract unusual diseases and disastrous complications.

715.   Don't get stressed out when you run a CODE. The patient is usually already dead. It's all up from here!

716.   Actual script of my most successful CODE in residency: (Visitor collapses pulseless in ICU)
        1) Tear his shirt off
        2) Put the pads on
        3) Clear
        4) Shock

717.   Avoid getting pinched in a tight spot. Don't get caught in the corner. Maintain degrees of freedom and look for a few ways out of any situation.

718. Most residencies are just long enough to teach you that rare things exist and that they never happen.

719. There is no hope for a resident who won't own their mistakes.

720. The intern's anxiety fades with their 4th year med student tan. But slower.

721. July is a great time to get sick with something rare. Eleven months later, the interns will assume you're just trying to get pain medicine.

722. The three greatest risks to the intern are:
      1) Depression
      2) Dehydration
      3) Cynicism

723. Announcement for the first of July: New interns, we don't mind your uncertainty! We need your humility, optimism and enthusiasm!!

724. The more people feel comfortable telling you what's going wrong with your patients the less goes wrong.

725. The first casualty of clinical education is common sense.

726. The wise resident departs any hospital floor at night asking the nurses: "Anything I can do for you before I leave?"

727. You do at least a hundred unnecessary things every day. When you stop doing them, you can work harder, longer, without getting as tired.

728. Knowing the lab or vital sign is half of it. Knowing which direction it's moving and how fast is the rest.

729. Never scoff at a patient who gets admitted repeatedly "for nothing." Everyone dies of something, eventually.

730. The most common resident lie: "I'll come back and we can talk about that later."

731. Learning medicine, we try cutting corners. In failing, we discover the ones that can't be cut.

732. The single most valuable trait in a medical trainee: Jolly persistence despite abject failure.

733. Medical Problem Solving Simplified:
    1. List the possibilities
    2. Rank them once by likelihood and once by deadliness
    3. Search for the ones at the top of both the lists
    4. Either find the diagnosis and treat it or exclude the most deadly and offer reassurance

734. By the end of your internship you have seen so much abnormal you have no idea what normal looks like. You aren't even normal anymore.

735. When I was a resident we used to say, "The later you stay, the later you stay."

736. You want to be perfect but you can't be perfect. You will have to accept being good enough and caring more.

737. As a physician in front of your patients it is your duty to remain in character. You are on stage with an audience who paid your to play your role.

738. Advice for interns starting in July: spend April, May, and June getting into the best shape of your life. Do your best not to lose it!

739. If you practice doctoring without compassion you may master it.

740. There are 13 Ways out of the Hospital:
    1) Discharge home
    2) Discharge to nursing home
    3) Discharge to hospice
    4) Discharge to street
    5) Discharge to friend or family member's home
    6) Discharge to rehab (physical or drug)
    7) AMA
    8) AWOL
    9) Discharge to jail
    10) Transferred to another hospital
    11) Sent to LTAC
    12) Died
    13) Always leave room for a miracle

741. Hang on tight to the dying patient by your teeth like a hungry dog but not so tight that you break the skin.

742. Nothing will improve your speed in the hospital like correctly identifying which problems are not your problems.

743. Right after you tell me, "I don't know," tell me how you are going to figure it out.

The Medical Educator

744. Nothing renews optimism in a cynical old doctor like brand new interns and medical students!

745. You can't teach it until you have mastered it. You can't master it until you teach it.

746. First learn to do the thing. Then figure out why you do it the way you do. Now you can teach it.

747. To win in the ring you must get hit in the gym.

748. All successes are resident successes. All failures are attending failures.

749. If you need help building a medical team, house staff team, or any team, watch Kurosawa's Seven Samurai.

750. Failing to correct a student's error is malice, not negligence.

751.   Med students need education. Interns need
        instruction. Residents need correction.
        Colleagues need inspiration.

752.   The bigger the crowd, the better the show.

753.   The moment you discover that something you've
        always said is wrong, stop saying it right away.

754.   Repetition is the foundation of learning. But
        don't forget:
        ☐   Repetition is the foundation of learning and
            also
        ☐   Repetition is the foundation of learning.

755.   Come quickly to the aid of sick patients in pain
        and dying who are trying to calm the guilt and
        fear of new trainees.

756.   Tell your students and residents to wear nice
        shoes to the hospital. You will look at them often
        as they stand on your shoulders.

757.   Never say something 100 times when you can
        just show it once.

758. With confidence, the student can accept criticism. Begin teaching by building confidence.

759. You can pin a lesson to the learner's brain with fear or laughter. Try laughter first.

760. A good teacher teaches you things you don't want to learn in a way you won't forget them until you discover they are true.

761. A satisfying academic career is an uneasy balance between seeing patients, teaching students and residents, and research & publishing. Oh yeah and
   - ☐ doing annoying administrative junk
   - ☐ trying to keep fit
   - ☐ spending time with family and friends
   - ☐ participating in your community
   - ☐ maintaining your emotional and spiritual condition
   - ☐ throwing tennis ball for dog

762. Med students are like kids at an orphanage. When you see one you like, adopt them. Once you have, stick with them through success and failure like you would your own kid.

763. Teaching (v.): Saying something that can't be forgotten. Don't say wrong things.

764. The best continuing medical education is done by exchanging stories with respected colleagues.

765. In the last few months before graduation, residents can only be taught by allowing them to make mistakes. Select them carefully.

766. Great teachers may be funny, shocking, dramatic, scary, upsetting, mystifying, charismatic or irritating. They cannot be boring.

767. It is easier to emulate than to spontaneously generate. Easier to follow a path than make one. The best trips are begun with guides. Find a mentor and try to follow their suggestions.

768. If you have lost your faith in medical education, attend a medical school graduation.

769. Good medical education is minimally repetitive for the learner and highly repetitive for the instructor.

770. Nothing pulls a house staff team together like
    1. Celebration of intern successes
    2. Humble ownership of failures by the attending

771. You can't ask a resident what they want to do for the patient before you decide what should be done.

772. If you spend some time in a dusty physical medical school library, you'll see that "modern medicine" is seamlessly connected to the ridiculous quackery of The Old Days.

773. You can't tell a resident or student how to own a mistake properly. You must show them.

774. Good teaching is like hammering a nail—good aim and repetition.

775. An academic doctor who can't inspire is a farmer without a plow. Seeds cast on unbroken ground will not germinate.

Mistakes and Errors

776. Errors in judgment must occur in the practice of an art which consists largely of balancing probabilities. —William Osler

777. For one mistake made for not knowing, ten mistakes are made for not looking. —JA Lindsay, MD, 1923

778. You should learn more from being wrong than being right.

779. Any deviation from standard care is sub-standard.

780. It's easier to criticize a good doctor than to be one.

781. If you must make a mistake, make sure it's big enough that someone finds it right away.

782. Don't miss a case of appendicitis that causes a positive urinalysis.

783. You are ten times more likely to make a mistake caring for the last patient of the day.

784. It's a rookie mistake not to call an experienced colleague when in doubt. Five minutes on the phone can save a lifetime of regret.

785. The best way to learn from your mistakes is to let somebody else make them.

786. Can't be taught who won't admit wrong.

787. The worst doctors will point out the errors of their colleagues; the best will tell you about their own. Thus you can differentiate them.

788. Don't worry about the mistake your colleague made today. Look for the ten you made.

789. The greatest teacher in the world is a disastrous mistake, recognized.

790. Nothing clouds medical judgment like guilt. Followed closely by the desire to get home at the end of the day.

791. You will be forgiven your ugly ignorance and imperfect judgment by performing this simple act of penance: Teach 10 doctors about each mistake you make.

792. "A man who has committed a mistake and doesn't correct it, is committing another mistake." —Confucius

793. Right now is the 2nd best time to find your mistake. The best time was 5 minutes ago.

794. I once told a patient "We need to discharge you from the hospital because there are sicker patients waiting to get in." It went over badly.

795. I once heard a resident say to a patient "We need to discharge you today because the hospital is a dangerous place." Never say that.

796. Nothing ensures your wrongness like your sureness.

797. Never do things no good doctor would do—you are better off making a mistake that everybody makes than a mistake nobody makes.

798. Hoping the new problem will go away before you have to figure it out sometimes works and never looks good.

799. At times a patient will die suddenly without warning. A careful review of nursing notes, vitals and labs will usually reveal the warning.

800. First guess is usually the best. Always make a list, though.

801. Practicing good medicine is hard. Avoiding bad outcomes is harder.

802. You spend your residency trying to learn to be right. You spend the rest of your career trying to learn not to be wrong.

803. You'd think the more doctors who agree about a diagnosis, the more right it is. In fact, the more that agree, the harder it is to convince any of them that they are wrong.

804. "I've been wrong before. I'll be wrong again." I say it to colleagues, nurses, patients and families. They need to know they are dealing with a human being, not a god.

805. In every diagnostic mystery, the physician chooses the error:
    a) Looked for deadly disease; didn't find it.
    b) Didn't look for deadly disease; patient died from it.

806. Some of the patients transferred to the MICU would have survived in their ward bed. The goal is not to have a patient die in a ward bed who would have survived in the MICU.

807. The patient's medical history you copy and paste from the last visit is usually mostly right. Hiding in there are legends and hearsay with no factual basis and a few bald-faced lies.

808. The only thing I hate worse than hearing from a colleague that I made a mistake is not hearing from my colleague that I made a mistake.

809. Usual care is optimal care. Any deviation from usual care is sub-optimal.

810. Pressing email "Reply All" is like kissing every girl at the wedding.

811. Try never to make a clinical decision without first deciding how you will fix it if you're wrong.

812. When lost, stop moving. Rushing in the wrong direction is worse than sitting still.

813. Your speed & efficiency comes from ignoring details. Your errors & mistakes come from ignoring details.

814. Checking for something and not finding it is not a mistake. Missing something important by not checking is a mistake.

815. If the doctor is at fault, the usual cause by specialty:
- ☐ Medicine: The Thing Not Done
- ☐ Surgery: The Thing Done Wrong

816. When reviewing a case where a patient dies in the hospital, you will find the early signs in changes of:
- vitals
- labs
- mental status

817. Loss of attention and failure of simple reminder systems are responsible for more medical errors than lack of brilliance.

818. Never do something you never do (if there is a more experienced operator available).

819. If you don't find your errors every day it's not because you aren't making them.

820. You become error-prone at the end of the day, the end of the week, the end of a stretch. Most especially the day before you start vacation.

821. The regretful doctor carries his shovel to the cemetery.

822. How To Make A Mistake:
    1. Make it honest
    2. Find it fast
    3. Take responsibility
    4. Apologize
    5. Figure out what you did wrong
    6. Never make it again
    7. Teach others not to make it

823. I learn nothing from Success. Failure is my professor, lecture and laboratory.

824. The young doctor can tell you with confidence what he knows. The old doctor can tell you with certainty what she does not know.

825. The only right response to being told you have made a mistake is "Thanks for letting me know."

826. The beauty of being a doctor is never making a mistake... that isn't immediately brought to your attention by three nurses and a pharmacist.

827.   Assuming the next one will be like the last one.

828.   Attributing all findings in the alcoholic to alcohol.

829.   Allowing patients who aren't sick to consume your time and energy.

830.   Ignoring an experienced nurse.

Malpractice: *Sometimes indicates bad practice. Always indicates hurt feelings.*

832. Write in the chart as if the patient and their family will read it. If things go badly, they will.

833. Some say they sue a doctor to make them better. I recommend they see the most-sued doctor they can find.

834. The physician does nobody a service by testifying on behalf of a plaintiff against another doctor.

835. More lawsuits come from not caring than not knowing.

836. You'll be wrong about half the time you think another doctor has made a mistake. The most critical among us are the least competent.

837. Plaintiff's attorneys love to ask, "Why didn't you order this inexpensive non-invasive test to rule out that life-threatening diagnosis?" It's often a very hard question to answer.

838. The more physicians are named in a lawsuit, the more likely none of them are guilty.

839. Once three doctors agree on the wrong diagnosis, the patient will die.

840. Even a lawyer can tell you how to make one "correct" medical decision. None could make the thousands you do each week.

841. Never let a physician whose signature is not in the chart make a medical decision for you when yours is.

842. More good doctors quit after being sued than bad ones.

843. Avoiding litigation involves sprinkling a little more kindness and compassion in the exam room and spilling a little more ink in the chart.

844. The story of many malpractice cases starts with the patient saying, "He didn't listen. He didn't care." Or the next doctor saying, "That never should have happened to you..."

845. Expert Witness: A doctor who has made the same error as the defendant but nobody noticed.

846. Dirt cleans off a lot easier than blood. —Maximus (Gladiator, movie, 2000)

847. Malpractice cases that are hard to win:
   1. One-legged lady
   2. Kid doesn't look right
   3. Guy will never work again

848. Your best notes will never become exhibits at trial.

849. A good malpractice case does not need negligence or causation. Big damages win big awards.

850. You best work leaves no trace. Your mistakes will be clear for the world to see in your notes, orders, and chart documentation.

851. When you testify as an expert against a fellow physician in a court of law, you do your colleague and your profession a disservice.

852. Learning to practice in a way that avoids bad outcomes is much harder than learning to practice good medicine. Ask any malpractice lawyer.

853. It's easier to defend "I made a list and picked the most likely diagnosis" than "I picked a diagnosis that I thought was likely."

854. The only "standard of care" in medicine is practice without negligence. —BMcC

855. Negligence: Failure to use reasonable ranges of medical judgment in the specific circumstances of this case at the time viewed prospectively. —BMcC

Burned Out

857.   Remember your purpose: You were put in this
        earth to heal the sick.

858.   When your compassion is low, the time spent
        with your dog should be high. Same when your
        compassion is high.

859.   They won't pay you enough to make you happy
        and nobody cares how hard you worked to get
        here.

860.   I don't know what they mean when they say
        "doctor, heal thyself" but get a dog.

861.   If your only choice is quit or die, quit. It doesn't
        have to be forever.

862.   When you feel you have no more to give,
        remember that while the patient is sick, you are
        merely tired. You have the luxury to heal the
        suffering!

863. What's the point of years of grueling medical education if the physician can't occasionally have a donut?

864. There is no greater treatment for your pains than to sit at the bedside and listen to the patient tell their story.

865. The only thing worse than your imperfect practice of medicine is you not practicing medicine. After setbacks, get back to work.

866. The best doctors learn to appreciate the easy cases because they leave time and energy for the hard ones.

867. If you love a person in medicine, you must occasionally tolerate them going out, acting a fool, drinking, blowing off steam, and raising a raucous rumpus. Bursting the restraints of clinical practice is an essential part of survival.

868.   Internal Medicine is an open-book test.

869.   Determining volume status is complicated and
        inexact. Don't obsess when faced with
        conflicting evidence. Remember you're usually
        just trying to establish the risk and benefit of a
        liter of saline or a single dose of Lasix.

870.   The diagnosis of shock is made by assessment of:
        1) The external appearance of the patient
            and
        2) The internal condition the physician
            looking at them.

871.   The best indication for testing for an aortic
        dissection is the thought, "I wonder if this patient
        has an aortic dissection?"

872.   There is no illness more serious than the one that
        causes the dry cleaning lady to close up her own
        shop and come to the hospital.

873. If the blood is missing, keep looking until you find the blood.

874. Don't fiddle with routine health care maintenance and outpatient medicines when you should be diagnosing the chief complaint. There will be no follow-up appointments if you can't keep them alive.

875. Not all tachycardic hypoxemic post-op patients with a normal CXR have a PE but not none of them do.

876. Nothing makes your differential diagnosis wronger than the discovery that the patient is pregnant.

877. Accident: Old guy falls down once. Illness: Old guy falls down more than once

878. Don't start checking blood tests and fishing for problems in the 99-year-old lady. Just get her back home before you screw something up.

879.   If you want to know why the patient is anemic, get the blood tests before you give the transfusion.

880.   The older you get, the more diseases you will die with. The number you die from stays about the same.

881.   Some doctors seem to magically know what to do next when a situation changes suddenly. It's because they thought about it yesterday.

882.   Not all fevers are caused by infections. Neither do all infections cause fever.

883.   A diagnosis for every medication and a medication for every diagnosis. This is how you check an admission H+P for accuracy.

884. Know at least 12 diagnoses for the differential of:
- o Tachycardia
- o Fever
- o Anemia
- o Weight loss
- o Nausea and vomiting
- o Chest pain
- o Elevated white blood cell count

885. Essential tools for the Internal Medicine Hospitalist: A decent pen, 3x5 index cards, a Sharpie, a chair, a smartphone and an Internet connection.

886. When a patient falls and breaks a hip, the internist's first question is, "Why did this person fall?"

887. The average person is born with excess bone marrow, hepatocytes and nephrons; insufficient cartilage, alveoli and neurons.

888. Any good internist loves to hear any story that starts with an age, a gender, and a symptom.

889. Some "spontaneous bacterial peritonitis" is really cholecyctitis, appendicitis, or diverticulitis. The worst cases are perforated viscus.

890. You can hide a big aortic dissection under the little words "rule out MI."

891. In Internal Medicine:
     o Your best guess is right about 85% of the time.
     o The unlikely diagnosis you have listed; 5%.
     o 10% of the time you haven't even considered the right diagnosis

892. You can't make a pulmonary infiltrate, a positive UA, or an abscess without white blood cells. But you can still make a fever.

893. There is nothing incidental about an asymptomatic renal cell carcinoma if it's found in your kidney.

894. Many people die after breaking a hip. Few of them die of a broken hip.

895. Young people get symptoms. Old people get confused.

896. In the elderly, confusion may be the sole presenting symptom of MI, sepsis, depression, appendicitis, hip fracture, hypoxia, impending death, it's getting late in the day, and natural progression of disease, among others.

897. The most valuable technological advance in the practice of Internal Medicine was the invention of the chair. For you to sit on. While you take a history .

898. Not all that wheezes is asthma.

899. Young and healthy get hot when they are infected. Old folks sometimes get cool. Room temperature even.

900. I know you read in the book that ischemic gut always gives you lactic acidosis but I've seen patients who didn't read the book.

901. Some cancers present with infection. Few infections present with cancer. Can you name them? (Start with HIV)

902. If you stick around long enough, you will come to respect compartment syndrome as a catastrophic complication you know nothing about. Ask your general or orthopedic surgery friends to tell you about it at lunch sometime.

903. Being a hospitalist is a great job not to have for 15 days a month.

904. You know you are an internist when you think, "My back hurts. Probably mets."

905. Most internists like baseball. It's slow as heck and you can talk the whole time. Orthopedic surgeons like football and ER doctors like hockey and basketball.

906. Sometimes Lasix makes the creatinine go down. Other times it makes it go up. Knowing the difference is Internal Medicine.

907.   Henoch-Schonlein purpura is a benign condition except when it causes perforations in the GI tract and rapid exsanguination or renal failure requiring dialysis.

908.   It may be a very atypical story for ACS but it's always a typical story for whatever it ends up being. Even if it ends up being ACS.

909.   You worry when a patient has a fever but worry more when the patient is heading toward room temperature.

910.   Elevated WBCs are interesting. Show me bands and I am listening close. Metamyelocytes and myelocytes and you have my full attention!

911.   If you are not sure if a hypotensive patient needs Lasix or saline, take a few minutes to transfer them to the MICU while you decide.

912. Common errors during long hospitalizations:
    1. Forgetting the chief complaint
    2. Dropping chronic problems from the problem list
    3. Missing trends in vitals and labs
    4. Ignoring medication side effects and drug-drug interactions
    5. Forgetting that this person once walked the earth, rode a bike, kissed their special someone goodnight

913. When take a history from a patient with chest pain, the first question to ask is "Why are you here?"

914. On the day you believe you have mastered medicine, you are ready to evaluate the patient with recurrent nausea and vomiting.

915. Like an egg half scrambled or a flip half flipped, some things can't be handed off at the end of a shift.

916. Everyone who loses weight without trying is sick with something.

917. Any disease that can cause a fever can cause a high fever. The height of the fever is no indication of the severity of illness causing it.

918. When you discover a 5cm lung mass, get a biopsy.

919. The patient who stops smoking for no specific reason may die soon.

920. Fever of unknown origin is New York City for internists. If you can make a diagnosis here, you can make it anywhere.

921. Elderly patients without fever or chills can still have infection as the source of their ills.

922. The diagnosis of shock is partly based on the appearance of the patient in the bed, vitals and labs. The rest is a feeling in the pit of your stomach.

923. Experience is a great teacher. Never let her teach you that young people:
   A. Never have heart attacks
   B. Never die of pneumonia.

924. The Two Essential Questions in Internal Medicine:
   1. Is this something or is it nothing?
   2. Is it more of the same or something new?

925. Subspecialty consultants have been known to famously miss diagnoses that are squarely located in the center of their daily practice.

926. Internal Medicine Hospitalists' Universal Answer: "I don't know, but I know a guy who does."

927. Proper treatment of chronic hypertension is often one of the most important things you can do. It's rarely the most important thing you can do today in the hospital.

928. An internist can run out of answers but she should never run out of questions. Diagnosis is accomplished by generating theories and testing them.

929. Never tell another doctor their diagnosis is wrong unless you can prove a better one.

930. Historically, internists have a gear-box like a farm tractor. The modern hospitalist has to have a close-ratio 6-speed like a racecar.

931. One of the joys of being a hospitalist is the feeling after some days off: "I want to go there again. I'm good at that job. They need me. I'm ready."

932. The 72 year old with a new headache every day for 3 weeks needs a head CT.

933. Show me unintentional weight loss or an albumin of 2 and I will show you a bonafide medical illness waiting to be diagnosed.

934. Every great internist is an angler, a gambler, and a boxer. They like to trick nature, be right and win against long odds. They don't give up and they don't get tired easily.

935. RED FLAGS for BACK PAIN: *Suggest there maybe something more serious than "musculoskeletal pain."*
   1. Fever
   2. Wakes from sleep
   3. No relief with rest
   4. Known cancer
   5. Focal neurological deficit
   6. Patient takes prednisone
   7. IVDA.

936. Medicine is more calculus than accounting. The present state of numbers is sometimes less important than their direction and rate of change.

937. PEA arrest is a two person CODE. One to run it and one to stand behind them whispering the differential diagnosis out loud off the card.

938. The human GI tract is like a personal computer. If it is not working properly, turn it off, wait awhile, and turn it back on.

939.   The patient with asthma who is not wheezing is either fine or nearly dead.

940.   When you see clubbing in COPD, look for another diagnosis. COPD does not cause clubbing.

941.   Oxygen is non-flammable. It only increases the flammability of flammable things. I was a chemistry major.

942.   Hypoxemia with a clear chest X-ray: A partial list
   1.   Asthma and COPD
   2.   Pulmonary embolus
   3.   CNS depression
   4.   OSA and OHS
   5.   Radiolucent foreign body
   6.   Don't forget hepatopulmonary syndrome!

943.   Pulmonologist (n.): A chess player who can play multiple boards at the same time. With some of the pieces on a ventilator.

944. Six things can fill alveoli:
  1) pus
  2) water
  3) blood
  4) cells
  5) protein and
  6) lipids. Yes, Smarty McSmarterton
  7) air

945. Sometimes the parapneumonic effusion is there on the day of admission and sometimes it shows up the 2nd or 3rd day.

946. It is essential to identify and drain empyema for two reasons:
  1. to prevent development of trapped lung and
  2. to speed recovery

947. Cats don't usually wear oxygen because they don't usually smoke.

948. COPD Rule of 20's:
  1. Takes about 20 pack/yrs to get COPD.
  2. About 20% of patients with COPD never smoked.

949. Have the patient with massive hemoptysis lie on their side with the healthy lung up so it can keep breathing while the sick one fills with blood.

950. The patient with severe pulmonary hypertension who is sick with anything may be about to die from it.

951. You can't deliver home oxygen to someone who lives in their car.

952. It's hard to scramble an egg in the bathroom but easy in the kitchen. It's hard to do critical care on the ward or elevator but easy in the ICU.

953. Yes, this patient has a history of asthma. Yes, this patient is hypoxic. It is not thus always true that this patient's hypoxia is a result of her asthma.

954.   Simultaneous bleeding and clotting is one of the
        most difficult clinical situations in medicine.

955.   A bone marrow biopsy hurts less if you tell the
        patient it's going to feel like a nurse standing on
        their butt cheek. On one foot. In heels.

956.   White blood cells go up and they go down.
        Sometimes it's something and sometimes it isn't.

957.   On our lovely Earth, god and nature created
        people dying of cancer and opium poppies. And
        doctors to introduce them to one another.

958.   The patient with multiple myeloma will likely die
        from kidney failure or infection before they die
        from multiple myeloma.

959. Three times your spleen will try to kill you:
1. Ruptures in MVA
2. Eats your platelets in ITP
3. Lets encapsulated organisms run wild when gone

960. When you consider ordering a fine needle aspiration of a lymph node, poke your own self with the needle then call a surgeon and ask for an <u>excisional biopsy</u>.

961. Lymphoma wants you to think all fevers are caused by infection.

962. When you tell a patient they have cancer, say "cancer" 10 times:
1. Cancer
2. Cancer
3. Cancer
4. Cancer
5. Cancer
6. Cancer
7. Cancer
8. Cancer
9. Cancer
10. Cancer. Then ask them what they have. About one time in ten they will say "cancer."

963. If you were "cured' with a nephrectomy for renal cell carcinoma 10 years ago and your back hurts, I'm looking for metastases from your renal cell carcinoma.

964. A hemoglobin of 7g/dL is a problem. A hemoglobin going from 15 to 7 in an hour is an emergency.

965. The CXR and UA show the white blood cells and the stuff that comes with them. A patient with no white blood cells can have a normal CXR and UA despite an infection.

966. Things that are not normal: nucleated RBC's in peripheral blood, an INR of 2 without ESLD or warfarin, PLTs of 20.

967. Oncologist (n.) v.1: A doctor who works side-by-side with Death every day but never speaks to him.

968. Oncologist (n.) v.2: A doctor who is trying to kill you more slowly than the cancer.

969.   The oncologist is the reason they put nails in coffins —Old Saying Among Physicians

970.   Some mean tumors come back after 10 years of remission: renal cell, breast, melanoma.

971.   The human body is forever trying to make a clot and dissolve a clot.

972.   Before beginning chemotherapy for cancer, establish a safe word with your oncologist.

Cardiology

973. There are 7 deadly causes of chest pain. Only one of them is "myocardial infarction." Know the other 6.

974. Ruling out MI doesn't tell you the cause of the patient's chest pain.

975. A stent in your coronary is like a magnet attracting stress tests, coronary angiograms and cardiologists to you evermore.

976. Digoxin used to be good medicine for rate control in atrial fibrillation and symptom relief in CHF.

977. Every once in a while, a patient will die of an MI a few weeks after a negative stress test. To teach you pathophysiology.

978. The anterior branch is the important one in the morbid anatomy of the coronary arteries. It may be called the artery of sudden death. —William Osler

979. The coronary artery is not a rigid metal pipe that gets clogged with calcium. It is a wriggling, constricting, dilating, clotting and lysing little worm.

980. Causes of CHF that can get better: Hypothyroid, alcoholic, peripartum CM, ischemic, viral myocarditis, Tako Tsubo.

981. A man is as old as his arteries. —Cazalis

982. Sandy Koufax's Sign: Ask the patient with chest pain to mime throwing a baseball. If their shoulder hurts, their problem is not their heart. It is their shoulder.

983. I am still waiting to read the case report of the patient whose life was saved by the low-fat low-salt cardiac hospital diet.

984. The chest pain of aortic dissection is also sometimes relieved with nitroglycerin.

985. The patient with aortic stenosis and syncope is running out of time.

986. Orthopnea has one of the shortest differential diagnoses. As far as I know, pulmonary edema is the only thing that reliably causes it.

987. Leg edema is *usually* a cosmetic issue. Unless it prevents the wearing of shoes. Or breaks down the skin causing cellulitis or ulcers.

988. One of the most reliable side effects in all of medicine is the headache that follows sublingual nitroglycerine.

989. DDX sinus tachycardia: Dehydration, bleeding, anemia, alcohol w/d, pain, hyperthyroid, PE, MI, valve failure, ESLD, meds, street drugs...

990. Most patients with chest pain would like to know they are not having a heart attack, but they also would like to know what they are having.

991. Cardiologists ruin more kidneys than nephrologists ruin hearts.

992. Cardiologist: An internist who thinks she can guess the right dose of furosemide better than you. Also, a life-saving stent/box-placer.

993. If your shoulder pain came on while you were shaking a shirt and now you can't lift your arm, it may not be your heart.

994. When an anesthesiologist notices "something funny" on the monitor, get a 12-lead EKG and a medical doctor.

995. Every day in America, thousands of patients can say, "They 'ruled out MI' but did nothing for the pain in my chest."

996. You'll never wish you could take back heparin so badly as when "rule out unstable angina" suddenly becomes "a clear case of aortic dissection."

997. Seven Deadly Causes of Chest Pain:
1. MI/USA
2. PE
3. Aortic dissection
4. Tension pneumothorax
5. Pericarditis with tamponade
6. Pneumonia
7. Boerhaave's or traumatic rupture of the esophagus
8. Pancreatitis
9. Peptic ulcer

998. The patient who dies soon after receiving SL NTG for chest pain may have had critical aortic stenosis.

999. You will know your diuresis is sufficient when your patient tells you about dreams of ice-cold lemonade.

Infectious Diseases: *Everybody calls them "ID"*

1000. If you haven't diagnosed syphilis, pertussis, HIV or TB lately, you've probably missed syphilis, pertussis, HIV and TB.

1001. Antibiotics make poor antipyretics.

1002. Blood cultures do not tell you your patient has bacteremia. They tell you your patient might have had bacteremia when the cultures were drawn.

1003. All fevers are intermittent.

1004. Getting the flu from a flu shot is like getting mauled by a bearskin rug.

1005. Fever in infection is rattle on the snake. Some bite without warning.

1006. Always startle when you see culture results with <u>gram-positive rods</u>: Listeria, Bacillus cereus, Clostridia, and Anthrax, among others.

1007. Tuberculosis mycobacteria are more like oysters who live stuck to rocks than fish who swim in the open sea. The AFB stain of pus or fluid can be negative followed by a positive biopsy of the serosa.

1008. Mycoplasma pneumonia is usually not a big deal but I saw a pregnant woman die from it.

1009. DDX leukocytosis: Infection, trauma, MI, leukemia, leukemia reaction, prednisone, cancer, post op, gout flare, bad day, and many others.

1010. Group least likely to refuse to immunize their kids: Immigrants to the US born in the developing world.

1011. All things in moderation, except antibiotics in bacterial meningitis.

1012. A Staph aureus UTI in an IV drug user may be a manifestation of endocarditis—via septic emboli to the kidneys.

1013. Endocarditis rarely causes chest pain. Not never.

1014. Intravenous drug users with endocarditis should not go home with central venous access.

1015. DDX fever: Infection, cancer, thrombosis, post op, connective tissue disease, drugs, hereditary (FMF), CNS injury, transfusion, TTP, HLH, and others.

1016. Courage (n): Not giving the patient antibiotics despite a high fever without a source.

1017. Folly (n): Not giving the septic patient antibiotics, early.

1018. Endotoxin is an excellent antihypertensive. A normal blood pressure in a patient who has always been high can be an early sign of sepsis.

1019. A good place to hide an infection is under a course of antibiotics started without a clear indication.

1020. God created Original Sin and Hevea brasiliensis to lessen its complications. (Look it up)

1021. ID doctors miss cancer more than oncologists miss infection.

1022. I worry less about a bad pneumonia with a high fever & high WBC count than one with no fever & a low WBC count.

1023. Bacteria are like cops. The good ones outnumber the bad ones. The bad ones spoil the reputation of the good ones.

1024. No matter what antibiotics a patient is receiving, there is always a hole. The list starts with Actinomyces and ends with Zoster.

1025. Two red legs is rarely bacterial cellulitis.

1026. Olser called vaccination among the greatest benefits conferred on mankind and offered to arrange funerals of anti-vaccination propagandists. Just so you know.

1027. Bacteria are generally not "good" or "bad." They are merely in good places or bad places. Except syphilis. And Neisseria gonorrhoeae. And...

1028. Only a few infectious diseases have nearly 100% *untreated* mortality:
    - Naegleria fowleri meningitis
    - Bacterial endocarditis
    - Rabies

1029. Show me two things most people don't have— like pneumonia and a septic hip—and I will show you a single disease.

1030. Diagnosis not to miss in the febrile returning traveller: Malaria. Especially falciparum. There are other ones too.

1031. You will hear someone say, "The fever and headache aren't meningitis because the patient's still alive a day later." They've never seen Listeria.

1032. Draw two circles that partly overlap. Label one "fever" and the other "infection." It's a Venn diagram. Study it carefully. Now go teach someone what you've learned.

1033. Staph epidermidis in the blood is not always a contaminant. It sometimes represents true bacteremia. Worry when:
    1) 2/2 cultures positive
    2) There is a potential source: surgical wound, device, endocarditis, central venous catheters, CNS shunt, and others
    3) It keeps showing up

1034. Clostridium difficile (n.): The new diagnosis that makes you wonder if that was really a UTI a week ago or just bacterial colonization.

1035. Infectious Disease Doctor (n.): An internist who can look things up faster than you who has friends in the lab and pharmacy.

1036. The strongest antibiotics will not save the febrile patient who is dying from a non-infectious cause of fever.

1037. Not all fevers are infection. Not all positive blood cultures are bacteremia. Still, fever plus positive blood cultures should make you think "BACTEREMIA!"

1038. Unless you have a time machine, it is ineffective to start with narrow antibiotics and broaden them in the face of treatment failure.

1039. An old man with a new back pain and a fever probably has vertebral osteomyelitis, discitis, and/or epidural abscess. Or some other bad thing.

1040. The patient with influenza will often remember the time on the face of the clock when the shaking chill first struck.

1041. You can lead a horse to water but you cannot keep an IV drug user from shooting narcotics into his PICC line.

1042. You will see influenza without fever and influenza without cough. And many fevers and coughs without influenza. It's a hard job.

1043. When I hear that some people do not vaccinate their kids for religious reasons, I am reminded that not all gods like children.

1044. Pseudomonas smells like grapes and Staph aureus looks like a bunch of grapes on a microscope slide. It's easier to remember things in pairs like this.

1045. Many people occasionally sweat at night. This is normal. When you have to get up and change your shirt or sheets, you have night sweats.

1046. The proper paradigm for all antibiotic treatment is to start broadly when treating empirically and narrow based on culture or serologic data.

1047. One third of human leprosy cases in the U.S. result from contact with armadillos. They live in Texas. Don't forget it.

1048. Measles is a mild self-limited viral infection in someone else's kid.

1049. It is a pervasive misconception in the lay population that osteomyelitis of the toe can be treated with topical over-the-counter antibiotic ointment.

1050. The most commonly encountered rabid animal in the U.S. is the raccoon. (2015)

1051. Ninety percent of diagnosis comes from the history. Yet, show me 2/2 positive blood cultures with Staph aureus and I don't care if he doesn't feel sick. He's sick.

1052. An ounce of prevention is worth a pound of cure, yet some patients with ascites would rather get a weekly paracentesis than take their diuretics.

1053. When you see hemoptysis in a patient with an artificial aortic graft, you may be nearly out of time.

1054. Never say, "It's not gut ischemia because the bicarbonate and lactate are normal."

1055. Traumatic rupture of the esophagus is not Boerhaave's. Boerhaave's is by definition spontaneous. This is usually irrelevant.

1056. There is no possible way on earth you could design a good study to prove that eating little seeds causes diverticulitis.

1057. The liver is a part of the immune system.
       Patients with chronic liver disease are universally
       immunosuppressed.

1058. The first sign of hepatic encephalopathy is day-
       night reversal. Unfortunately perfect for a
       drinking life.

1059. I once met a man who used to have his ascites
       drained once a week. Now he walks about,
       taking no medicine. It's not a miracle. The liver
       has some capacity to regenerate.

1060. Gastroparesis is exclusively a complication of
       diabetes except in the substantial percentage of
       patients who have gastroparesis without
       diabetes.

Rheumatology: *The easiest elective for students and residents but a really hard job in real life!*

1061. A patient with lupus who has a new symptom is usually suffering another complication of lupus. Or its treatment.

1062. Race is rarely relevant in a patient's history. One exception: A "young Hispanic woman with lupus" should get your attention every time.

1063. A young female patient with lupus and chest pain may have a heart attack and she may have a pulmonary embolus. Miss neither.

1064. When you order a "sed rate" (ESR), you are putting up the white flag that says "I don't know!" Or you're looking for PMR. Or you're a rheumatologist. Or you are following a chronic infection like osteomyelitis.

Addiction

1065.   Alcohol is safe for those who drink normally. The rest it kills without mercy at a young age.

1066.   Do not try to frighten the alcoholic with the threat of dying. He is not afraid of dying. He is afraid of living. —Chuck C.

1067.   "Definition of an alcoholic: A patient who drinks more than their doctor." —Popular Wisdom, incorrect

1068.   You need not drink every day to be an alcoholic. Nor to die as one.

1069.   Many people are a shot of heroin away from a lifetime of opiate addiction.

1070.   Addicts choose addiction like kids choose to have diabetes.

1071. "Substance abuse" is a misnomer. Is there a more appropriate use for heroin than fending of symptoms of heroin withdrawal?

1072. No matter how bad an alcoholic looks to you, the world looks worse to him when the drink wears off.

1073. Alcoholism is an arithmetic disability: The inability to keep count after the first drink.

1074. Telling an addict to stop using is like telling a patient with lymphoma to stop having cancer.

1075. Advice from a 65-year-old patient: "Never start smoking the crack cocaine. It's very addictive."

1076. Some alcoholics dislike AA. Some people with cancer dislike chemotherapy. Avoiding unpleasant treatment is a luxury reserved for the healthy and those willing to die unnecessarily.

1077. One person who doesn't get better with practice is the alcoholic with drinking.

1078. Don't say, "You need to stop drinking or you will die." Would you ever say, "You need to stop having melanoma or you will die"?

1079. Frequency of drinking does not identify the alcoholic. Loss of control after the first drink and bad consequences do.

1080. The worst thing that can happen to an alcoholic is occasional bouts of normal, controlled drinking. Second worse: A spouse who insists he's not an alcoholic.

1081. The alcoholic who prioritizes drink over food is neither stupid nor insane. He is making a rational decision to survive.

1082. The best way to kill an alcoholic is to tell him "I don't think you're an alcoholic." The second best way is to tell him you think he can get sober on his own.

1083. For an alcoholic, the bottle is an emotional credit card. He can put off feeling pain today but the bill comes back with interest tomorrow.

1084. If a patient tells you his favorite drink is vodka, his chance of being an alcoholic is doubled. If mouthwash or hand sanitizer, tripled.

1085. You scare an alcoholic much more when you tell him he can't drink again than when you tell him he is going to die.

1086. A sober alcoholic can sometimes reach a suffering alcoholic when no doctor ever could.

1087. That which does not kill you makes you stronger. Except tequila.

1088. The most common treatment for alcohol withdrawal is alcohol. This is why most towns have bars and liquor stores that open first thing in the morning.

1089. Alcohol makes weak men feel strong and eventually makes strong men weak.

1090. Some doctors discharge patients with alcohol withdrawal with benzodiazepines so they can get sober at home. This never helps but most alcoholics love to experiment with them.

1091. Telling the alcoholic not to drink is like telling the tornado not to spin. If you want to help, give directions to the storm cellar.

1092. For the alcoholic to stop drinking, the alcoholic must die. Into his lifeless body, a sober man may be born.

1093. Your best disappointed schoolmarm face and wagging finger have never gotten an alcoholic sober. Not even once.

1094. The people who try hardest to keep count of their drinks are the worst at it.

1095. Most friends of an alcoholic will tell you he drinks normally. Because most alcoholics keep only alcoholics as friends.

1096. For the alcoholic, drinking is usually not a
       problem. It is a solution to problems.

Nephrology: *We call the kidneys "the beans." Because of the shape.*

1097. The only thing keeping the ~7 billion human beings on Earth from having acute renal failure today was a) thirst and b) free access to water, yesterday.

1098. Nephrologist: A smart internist armed with a calculator who is usually right. When she's wrong she has a machine that will fix everything.

1099. The kidney is smarter than you but only if you give it enough salt and water to work its magic.

1100. The half-life of insulin is increased in patients with end stage renal disease thus resulting in some patients who are "cured of diabetes" around the time they start dialysis. Insulin is metabolized in the glomerulus somewhere.

1101. "Hematuria" without red cells: (Things that cause red pee)
    o Myoglobinuria (rhabdomyolysis)
    o Rifampin
    o Beets
    o Really dry

1102. You want to see eosinophils in the urine in AIN. Old books say you will see them. You don't always see them.

1103. A banana has about 1mEq K+ per inch. One banana = ~10mEq potassium. —Stu Linas, MD

1104. Irrespective of the cause of acute renal failure or their chief complaint upon presentation to the hospital, patients on chronic hemodialysis usually die of a heart attack.

1105. There are 7 classes of antihypertensives. Each one will bring the SBP down about 10mmHg. A patient with a systolic blood pressure of 210mmHg may need all 7.

1106. The kidney is usually smart about salt and water, but gets dumber when there is a tumor in the brain or lung.

1107. If the patient has a dialysis catheter and a fever there may be an infection somewhere else besides the dialysis catheter.

1108. Around the time the patient with ESRD starts HD, diabetes will require less insulin and lupus may improve. That's all the good news I have.

1109. It's usually a little easier to get water in the human body than to get it out.

1110. Some people live more than 10 years after starting hemodialysis for ESRD. That's about 365 times longer than without.

1111. The single most valuable renal-protective therapy is an intact thirst mechanism and free access to water.

Endocrinology

1112. Adrenal insufficiency may present with "acute abdomen and sepsis" or hyponatremia and hyperkalemia. The patient does not need to show all the features of adrenal insufficiency to have it. It's a spectrum disease.

1113. Doctors with diabetes are often good at managing their blood sugar. They are not necessarily good at managing patient's blood sugars.

1114. People don't get foot ulcers looked at early because they are afraid of losing their foot. As a result, they lose their foot.

1115. People with diabetes hide things in their socks. Like the cause of death.

1116. Patients normally on insulin who are NPO should have D5 in their IV fluids. They eat carbohydrates every other day of their life, right?

Neurology and Psychiatry: *Brain stuff*

1117. Neurologist (n.): You know how it's easy for an orthopedic surgeon to diagnose a broken bone and fix it? The opposite of that.

1118. Suicide is a complication of untreated depression like a heart attack is a complication of untreated hypertension.

1119. When an old man gives away his dog he's going to kill himself. My dad did this.

1120. It's not a normal neurological exam unless the patient can get out of bed and walk across the room.

1121. The patient can no more will away the hopeless despair of depression than he can repair his own aortic dissection.

1122. It may help you understand the suicidal to know they have made a decision to murder their kidnapper and tormentor.

1123. I don't care what you saw in anatomy lab or read on the chest CT, emotional pain is substernal.

1124. Nobody can stop someone from killing themselves if they are dead set on it.

1125. Benzodiazepines can treat and cause delirium. In the same patient.

1126. It's fine to seize the day, but if you are supposed to take valproic acid, take that too.

1127. Any person who lives alone with >3 cats has a diagnosis.

The Emergency Department: *Don't call it "the emergency room" even if it's only one room.*

1128. Places you can hide a unit of blood:
    1) Chest: pleural space
    2) Belly: peritoneal space, gut lumen, retroperitoneal
    3) Extremity: long bone or pelvic fracture
    4) The street: the accident scene.

1129. The patient who returns to the ER for the 3rd time in 48 hours will usually get admitted and it's usually right.

1130. If you invented a naloxone for ethanol, you would be the richest person in the whole world. Then you would go bankrupt from lawsuits.

1131. Be nice to the people you know. They are much more likely to kill you than complete strangers.

1132. After 6 hours, for every hour a patient spends in the ED the chance that anyone knows what the hell is wrong with them drops by 10%.

1133. General Surgeon (n.): For some, suffering is a vocation.

1134. One time I gently nudged the bed with my knee and the patient grabbed his stomach and winced in pain. I said "call the surgeon." Within a few days, that patient had been transfused more than 100 units of blood for GI bleeding from Henoch Schonlein Purpura (HSP).

1135. Acute abdomen (n.): The belly possessed by a patient who feels so bad that they will consent to anything.

1136. The only people allowed to give Lasix for edema without having a diagnosis to explain it are surgeons.

1137. Surgeons don't cause infections, bacteria do. It makes them feel better when you tell them this.

1138. Most patients on high blood pressure medicines don't need them for the first couple of days after surgery. Surgeons and anesthesiologists know this better than internists.

1139. Nobody may know why this patient is on 100mcg fentanyl patch, but hopefully everybody knows the post-op period is the worst time to discontinue it.

1140. In the elderly, a long bone or pelvic fracture can be a hematologic, cardiac and vascular event as well as an orthopedic one.

1141. The aged male prostate is a sensitive detector of pain, medications, inactivity, illness, and anxiety.

1142. Even a small operation performed in the operating theater would usually count as a decent stab wound in the emergency department.

1143. Stethoscope (n.): A rubber & metal indicator that allows an orthopedic surgeon to quickly identify a hospitalist when a patient develops a non-bony problem.

1144. General surgery resident's two standard answers to everything:
   1. Call me back if he gets sicker.
   2. Why didn't you call me sooner?

1145. The cold pulseless foot is a medical emergency like an ST elevation MI.

1146. What do you call a chatty general surgical intern? Future ED doctor.

1147. Many people wait longer than I would to seek help when they have a foot ulcer exposing the skeleton.

1148. It takes about five years after residency for a good surgeon to learn when not to operate. The bad ones never learn.

1149. Show me a cold, pulseless foot and I will show you a surgeon. Right away.

1150. Pray each morning that you will lay your head down at night still a good operative candidate.

1151.   Sometimes the foot with critical limb ischemia hurts and sometimes it finally stops hurting for the first time in months.

1152.   One commonly used test for bone density is the ladder.

1153.   A good surgeon is not a power saw who cuts when you pull the trigger. A good surgeon is a physician who can tell you if an operation is necessary.

1154.   All kinds of doctors will tell you a patient needs an operation. Only a surgeon can tell you a patient doesn't need an operation.

Colleagues and The Other Specialties

1155. Don't waste time asking a bunch of stupid questions on the phone. Go see the patient.

1156. A good radiologist can save you from a bad surgeon. A good surgeon can save you from a bad radiologist.

1157. ID doctors are afraid of cats. Pulmonologists; birds. Internists; babies. ER doctors; nothing.

1158. A good surgeon thinks 20 steps ahead. A good hospitalist thinks 20 days ahead. A good family medicine doctor thinks 20 years ahead.

1159. In nature, human childbirth is a completely normal and natural process with a tragically high mortality for both mother and infant.

1160. When an internist says a patent is crashing it's not like when an OB says a patient is crashing.

1161. Collegiality among physicians is as essential as medical knowledge.

1162. Pediatricians get paid like schoolteachers. I guess because they get the privilege of spending their days with febrile infectious screaming kiddos and their patience-stretching parents.

1163. Never take care of a diagnosis that you never take care of. Practicing outside your scope of practice is indefensible.

1164. Pulmonologists never own pet birds but cardiologists eat chilidogs and trauma surgeons own guns.

1165. Emergency Medicine Doctor (n.): America's Urban Primary Care Provider.

1166. Family Medicine Doctor: The right doctor to tell your symptoms to at a cocktail party.

1167. Pathologist (n.): A doctor who is never proven wrong by the clock or calendar

1168. Interventional Radiologist (n.): A surgeon who will close your incision with a Hello Kitty Band-Aid.

1169. Internists treat some problems caused by patients' own bad decisions. Pediatricians; by parents. OBs; it's always some guy.

1170. Every Hospitalist needs three good friends: 1) A good general surgeon, 2) A good radiologist, 3) A good pathologist. A good pharmacist and social worker won't hurt, either!

1171. Never take care of a diagnosis that you never take care of. Practicing outside your scope of practice is indefensible.

1172. Surgery (noun): A stressful procedure designed to manifest and exacerbate existing medical problems

1173. A smart surgeon will keep an internist around as a good luck charm to keep post-op patients alive.

1174. Your colleague may be confident and cavalier at the curbside but she will become suddenly uncertain and worried when formally consulted.

1175. A physician who has never seen your patient can add to your differential diagnosis. Never let them subtract from it.

1176. A good surgeon is a doctor who can operate and knows when not to operate. —Theodor Kocher (1841–1917)

1177. An ER doctor is a physician who can make the right decisions, fast, and sometimes even for the right reasons.

1178. Dentist (n.): Never happy to see one. More unhappy if you don't.

1179. Veterinarian (n.): A pediatrician who gets paid in cash.

1180. Anesthesiologist (n.): The most important doctor you will never remember.

1181. An internist is a doctor who looks at a chess board of a half finished game and likes to try to figure out how to win both sides.

1182. You know you are a family medicine doctor when you think, "My back hurts. Never mind there are 50 patients in the waiting room."

1183. You know you are an orthopedic surgeon when you think, "My back hurts. I am 50. Time to retire!"

1184. You know you are an anesthesiologist when you think, "My back hurts. I wonder if it's the horse or the jet ski?"

1185. You know you are a radiologist when you think, "My back hurts. God I hate people who order plain films for back pain."

1186. You know you are a transplant surgeon when you think, " My back hurts. Since when do gods have pains?"

1187. You know you are a nephrologist when you think, "My back hurts. But at least I am still making good urine. Avoid NSAIDS."

1188. You know you are an ID doctor when you think, "My back hurts. Probably vertebral osteomyelitis, discitis, and an epidural abscess. Maybe an atypical mycobacterium. I wish I was a hospitalist."

1189. You know you are a cardiologist when you think, "My back hurts. I should take the Porsche tomorrow."

1190. You know you are a pediatrician when you think, "My back hurts. Why do I have to keep explaining to people that vaccines don't cause autism?"

1191. You know you are a palliative care doctor when you think, "My back hurts. DNR, MS Contin, Zofran, Ativan, visit from therapy dog."

1192. You know you are an OB/GYN when you think, "My back hurts. Every day since the first day of my internship."

1193. You know you are an ICU doctor when you think, "My back hurts. It's probably nothing until I am on 3 pressors."

1194. You know you are a neurologist when you think, "My back hurts. Call me back after you get the MRI."

1195. You know you are a plastic surgeon when you think, "My back hurts. B ut my jawline looks like a Greek statue."

1196. You know you are a psychiatrist when you think, "My back hurts. Is it okay to talk to myself about it?"

Great Quotes from the History of Medicine

There is really no genius to this project. I started by reading all the great quotes by all the famous old dead doctors I could find. And my two favorite living aphorism authors: Clifton Meador, MD and Moshe Schein, MD. After awhile, I started to see through the formula or sparkle that separated the pearls from the pebbles. Few of my aphorisms floated in from sky. Many are variations and iterations of other brilliant words by doctors far more brilliant than me. Here are some of them. You will see below that the formula is not exclusive to medicine but extends to great thinkers in religion and politics and clever authors of all types. While I have done my best to properly attribute these quotes, you quickly learn in this realm that imitation and straight theft are nothing new. William Osler, a high producer of original pithy statements, often repeated the words of others without attribution. All this is to say I have done my best to figure out who said it first but there are surely errors for which I apologize beforehand. If you are pretty sure your facts are straighter than mine, send me an edit at medicalaxioms@gmail.com.

The lesser the indication, the greater the complication. —William Halsted, MD (1852-1922)

The lesser the indication, the greater the complication. —Mark M. Ravitch (1910-1989)

Young men kill their patients; old men let them die. —James Gregory (1753-1821)

Never be the first but never be the last to accept change. —Angus B. McLachlin (1908-1987)

Never believe what a patient tells you his doctor has said. —Sir William Jenner (1815-1898)

A surgeon maintains a mental catalogue of the things he did wrong at various times in his career and tries never to repeat them. —F. Moore

Teach thy tongue to say "I don't know." —Maimonides b. 1135

Don't think, just do. —Horace, b.65 BC

All who drink of this remedy recover in a short time, except those whom it does not help, who all die. —Galen, ~100 AD

It is difficult to make the asymptomatic patient feel better. —Stanley O. Hoerr (1909-1990)

It is much more important to know what sort of a patient has a disease than what sort of a disease a patient has. —William Osler

Do not hesitate to admit failures, as they must show the mode and places of improvement. —Theodor Billroth (1829-1894)

The best of healers is good cheer. —Pindar b. 522 BC

Never lose sight of the end and object of all your studies; the cure of disease and the alleviation of suffering. —William Osler

Don't think. Thinking is the enemy of creativity. You can't try to do things. You simply must do things. —Ray Bradbury

The fact that your patient gets well does not prove that your diagnosis was correct. —Samuel J. Meltzer

To teach is to learn twice. —Joubert, 1842

There is no higher mission in this life than nursing God's poor. — William Osler, in Aequanimitas

A surgeon is judged by three A's: ability, availability and affability. — Paul Rexnikoff (1896-1984)

Old persons are sometimes as unwilling to die as tired-out children are to say good night and go to bed. —Joseph Sheridan Le Fanu

Next to being right in this world, the best of all things is to be clearly and definitely wrong... —Thomas Henry Huxley

We keep moving forward opening new doors and doing new things, because we're curious and curiosity keeps leading us down new paths. —Walt Disney

One of the greatest satisfactions one can ever have comes from the knowledge that he can do some one thing superlatively well. — Odlum

Three things in human life are important: the first is to be kind; the second is to be kind; and the third is to be kind. —Henry James

Greatness is usually the result of a natural equilibrium among opposite qualities. —Diderot, 1761

Abandon hopeless projects early. —Mark Reid, MD

Next to the promulgation of the truth, the best thing I can conceive that a man can do is the public recantation of an error. —J. Lister

A consultant is a man sent in after the battle to bayonet the wounded. —Fred Metcalf

When a lot of remedies are suggested for a disease, that means it cannot be cured. —Anton Chekhov

Any theory is better than no theory. —Fuller Albright.

The first report of any new operation is rarely unfavorable. —Mark M. Ravitch (1910-1989)

A good surgeon is a doctor who can operate and knows when not to operate. —Theodor Kocher (1841-1917)

More is missed by not looking than by not knowing. —Tomas McCrae, b. 1870

I hear and I forget. I see and I remember. I do and I understand. — Confucius

The feasibility of an operation is not the best indication for its performance. —Lord Cohen Henry

Never go to a doctor whose office plants have died. —Erma Bombeck.

When I do good, I feel good. When I do bad, I feel bad. That's my religion. —Abraham Lincoln

Better to remain silent and be thought a fool than to speak out and remove all doubt. —Abraham Lincoln

Look wise, say nothing, and grunt. Speech was given to conceal thought. —William Osler

The amount of narcotic you use is inversely proportional to your skill. —Martin H. Fischer, b.1879

Medicine is a science of uncertainty and an art of probability. — William Osler, MD

Chance favors the prepared mind. —Louis Pasteur

Bedside manners are no substitute for the right diagnosis. —Alfred P. Sloan, Jr.

To do great work one must be very idle as well as very industrious. —Samuel Butler

You can do very little with faith, but you can do nothing without it. —Samuel Butler, The Note Books of Samuel Butler

Prayer indeed is good, but while calling on the gods a man should himself lend a hand. —Hippocrates

Don't believe everything you hear. But don't ignore it, either. — Horace Reid, Jr. (my dad)

It is as important to know what sort of person has the disease as to know what sort of disease the person has. —Caleb Parry, b. 1755

Continuous eloquence is tedious. —Pascal, 1670

In the sick room, ten cents' worth of human understanding equals ten dollars' worth of medical science. —Martin H. Fischer

No families take so little medicine as those of doctors, except those of apothecaries. —Oliver Wendell Holmes

Once you've tried everything and all hope is lost, try stopping everything. —Kevin Martin, MD

In no relationship is the physician more often derelict than in his duty to himself. —William Osler

Soap and water and common sense are the best disinfectants. — William Osler from *Sir William Osler : Aphorisms from His Bedside Teachings and Writings.* (1961) edited by Robert Bennett Bean

Common sense in matters medical is rare, and is usually in inverse ratio to the degree of education. —William Osler

Lord, deliver me from the man who never makes a mistake, and also from the man who makes the same mistake twice. —William J. Mayo, MD

It is much easier to add drugs than to subtract them. —Stephen J. Prevoznik

Let your entrance into the sick room decrease, not increase, the irritability of your patient. —Martin H. Fischer, MD

"Any theory is better than no theory." —Fuller Albright, noted endocrinologist, b. 1900

That which can be foreseen can be prevented. —Dr. William J. Mayo

Your thoughts become words. Words become actions. Actions become habit. Habits become character. Character becomes destiny. –Laozi

I prefer to be called a fool for asking the question rather than remain in ignorance. —John Homans, 1872

The way to heal is through cold steel. —Richard B. Fratianne, MD

Your patient didn't read the textbook. —Rebecca Tuetken, MD PhD

To each one of you the practice of medicine will be very much as you make it. —William Osler

The treatment of a disease may be entirely impersonal, the care of a patient must be completely personal. —Francis W. Peabody, MD

The dumbest kidney is smarter than the smartest doctor. —Anonymous

Restlessness is discontent and discontent is the first necessity of progress. Show me a thoroughly satisfied man and I will show you a failure. —Thomas A. Edison

Begin early to make a threefold category--clear cases, doubtful cases, mistakes. And learn to play the game fair... —William Osler

It takes considerable knowledge just to realize the extent of your own ignorance. —Thomas Sowell

"Show me a young beautiful cocaine addict and I will show her the door." —Oscar London.

Create the illusion of being less stressed than your patients. —Oscar London.

It is much easier to make a wrong diagnosis than it is to unmake it.
—Francis W. Peabody, MD

We palliate what we cannot cure. —Samuel Johnson, 1755

The most important result of any surgical operation is a live patient.
—Charles H. Mayo

He who works with his hands is a labourer. He who works with his
head and his hands is a craftsman. —St. Francis of Assisi

If we cannot be clever, we can always be kind. —Sir Alfred Fripp,
British surgeon b. 1865

He who studies medicine without books sails an uncharted sea, but
he who studies medicine without patients does not go to sea at all.
—Osler

The incision must be as long as necessary and as short as possible.
—Theodor Kocher

The basic guideline is "would you have this done to yourself, your wife, your child, your parent?" —Mark M. Ravitch

Ninety percent of this game is half-mental. —Yogi Berra

The greater the ignorance, the greater the dogmatism. —William Osler.

It's not the size of the dog in the fight, it's the size of the fight in the dog. —Mark Twain

A surgeon maintains a mental catalogue of the things he did wrong at various times in his career and tries never to repeat them. —Francis D. Moore

A patient who says he must borrow money to pay you will borrow the money, but won't pay you. —J. Chalmers Da Costa

"If it fails, admit it frankly and try another. But above all, try something." —Franklin D. Roosevelt

Walking is the best possible exercise. Habituate yourself to walk very far. —Thomas Jefferson.

When someone is giving you his opinion, you should receive it with deep gratitude even though it is worthless. –Yamamoto Tsunetomo, (early 18th century) from Hagakure The Book of the Samurai

A man who has never once erred is dangerous. –Yamamoto Tsunetomo

A good surgeon is a doctor who can operate and knows when not to operate. —Theodor Kocher (1841–1917)

Young men kill their patients; old men let them die. —James Gregory

The progress of disease is not suspended between 5 pm and morning rounds. —Mark M. Ravitch

Whether you think you can, or you think you can't, you're right. — Henry Ford

It is an unpardonable mistake to go about among patients with a long face. —William Osler, Aequanimitas

The patient is always more anxious to talk than to listen. —Theodor Billroth

The more I practice the luckier I get. —Arnold Palmer, inventor of a delicious warm-weather beverage and golfer

He who can discriminate between the possible and the impossible is the wisest physician. —Herophilus

Next to being right in this world, the best of all things is to be clearly and definitely wrong. —Huxley

Common sense in medical matters is rare and is usually in inverse ration to the degree of education. —Osler

Patients should have rest, food, fresh air, and exercise "the quadrangle of health." —William Osler

Never believe what a patient tells you his doctor has said. —Sir William Jenner

You can't live a perfect day without doing something for someone who will never be able to repay you. —John Wooden

You can easily judge the character of a man by how he treats those who can do nothing for him. —Malcolm S. Forbes.

Me as a kid: "Mom, where's my [whatever thing]?
My mom: "It's wherever you had it last."
(Note: This was 100% correct)

The treatment of a disease may be entirely impersonal; the care of a patient must be completely personal. —Francis W. Peabody

A good heart and kidneys can survive all but the most willfully incompetent fluid regimen. —Mark M. Ravitch, MD

It is difficult to make the asymptomatic patient feel better. — Stanley O. Hoerr

The last man to see the necessity for re-operation is the man who performed the operation. —Mark M. Ravitch, MD

Punctuality is the prime essential of the physician. If invariably on time, he will succeed even in the face of professional mediocrity. — William Osler

Bury the past and start afresh today with the firm resolve to waste not an hour of the short and precious time which is before you. — William Osler

Never let your tongue say a slighting word of a colleague. —WS Thayer in Osler the Teacher, in Osler and Other Papers, 2.

One special advantage of the skeptical attitude of mind is that a man is never vexed to find that after all he has been in the wrong. – William Osler

Do not hesitate to admit failures, as they must show the mode and places of improvement. —Theodor Billroth (1829–1894)

Definition of a double blind trial: two orthopaedic surgeons trying to read an electrocardiogram. —Nick J. Taffinder

You can't always be clever, but you can always be kind. —Charles Wilson Moran

All that we are is the result of what we have thought. The mind is everything. What we think we become. —Buddha

Skin is the best dressing. —Joseph Lister

There is nothing so cruel as ignorance. –Gull, 1923

For every complex problem there is an answer that is clear, simple, and wrong. —H.L. Mencken

Marriage is a wonderful institution, but who would want to live in an institution... —H.L. Mencken

Never lose sight of the end and object of all your studies; the cure of disease and the alleviation of suffering. —William Osler

Don't pile up money for your children. Give them the best education possible, and let them make their own way. —Blanche Ebbutt, 1913

If you're not planning for failure, you're not planning. —Seth Trueger

Never believe what a patient tells you to the detriment of a brother physician even though you may think it to be true. —William Osler

He who has a why to live can bear almost any how. —Friedrich Nietzsche

A witty saying proves nothing. —Voltaire b. 1694 (as read on my Good Earth tea bag tag)

A goal properly set is halfway reached. —Zig Ziglar

Experience is fallacious and judgment difficult. —Hippocrates as quoted in Oslers 4th edition of Principles and Practice of Medicine

Everything has been said before, but since nobody listens we have to keep going back and beginning all over again. —Andre Gide, 1891

Cure sometimes, treat often, comfort always. —Hippocrates

The purpose of human life is to serve, and to show compassion and the will to help others. —Albert Schweitzer

The genius rarely makes a successful practitioner. —William Osler.

A physician who treats himself has a fool for a patient. —William Osler

Our prime purpose in this life is to help others. And if you can't help them, at least don't hurt them. —Dalai Lama

Shut up at once the patient who would tell you of the faults of a professional brother. They will go to another and say the same of you. —William Osler

Children are not little adults but paediatricians are. —Christopher Williams, b. 1938

Many disputes in medicine arise as a result of "a convenient forgetfulness of our own failings." —William Osler

The physician is Nature's assistant. —Galen

A diagnosis is easy as long as you think of it. —Soma Weiss, MD, b. 1899

What we call experience is often a dreadful list of ghastly mistakes. —J. Chalmers Da Costa, Surgeon and writer, (1863–1933)

The medical profession is a noble and pleasant one, though laborious and often full of anxiety. —Andrew J. Symington (1825-1898)

The best way to destroy an enemy is to make him a friend. —Abraham Lincoln

Do not think that love has to be extraordinary. What we need is to love without getting tired. —Mother Teresa

It is the enemy who can truly teach us to practice the virtues of compassion and tolerance. —Dalai Lama

Have compassion for all beings, rich and poor alike; each has their suffering. Some suffer too much, others too little. —Buddha

If you want others to be happy, practice compassion. If you want to be happy, practice compassion. —Dalai Lama

Prayer indeed is good, but while calling on the gods a man should himself lend a hand. —Hippocrates, ~400 BC

Fear leads to anger. Anger leads to hate. Hate leads to suffering. — Yoda.

If it sounds good, it is good. —Duke Ellington

Foolish is the doctor who despises the knowledge acquired by the ancients. —Hippocrates

Leave nothing to chance, overlook nothing; combine contradictory observations and allow yourself enough time. —Hippocrates

He who desires to practice surgery must go to war. —Hippocrates

Use strengthens. Disuse debilitates. —Hippocrates, b. 460BC

Doctors are the best-natured people in the world, except when they get fighting each other. —Oliver Wendell Holmes, b. 1809

In teaching the medical student the primary requisite is to keep him awake. —Chevalier Jackson b. 1865

A man is as old as his arteries. —Thomas Sydenham.

It is the duty of a doctor to prolong life. It is not his duty to prolong the act of dying. —Lord Horder, 1936

A surgeon should have three diverse properties: 1) heart of a lion, 2) eyes of a hawk, and 3) hands of a woman. John Halle (1529–1568) [paraphrased]

It's not that I'm so smart, it's just that I stay with problems longer. —Albert Einstein

There are only two ways to live your life. One is as though nothing is a miracle. The other is as though everything is a miracle. —Einstein

We are like dwarves perched on the shoulders of giants. —Bernard of Chatres. 12th century, AD

The expectations of life depend upon diligence; the mechanic that would perfect his work must first sharpen his tools. —Confucius

Never give a sword to a man who can't dance. —Confucius

Our greatest glory is not in never falling, but in rising every time we fall. —Confucius

Choose a job you love, and you will never have to work a day in your life. —Confucius

When you are laboring for others let it be with the same zeal as if it were for yourself. —Confucius

Fair average abilities, well used, often carry their owner above the heads of abler men. —William Osler.

Never lie. —George Washington (attributed)

Verily I say unto you, Inasmuch as ye have done it unto one of the least of these my brethren, ye have done it unto me. —Jesus

DIY Index: Write your favorites down here

DIY Index: Write your favorites down here

DIY Index: Write your favorites down here

Made in the USA
Middletown, DE
17 August 2018